Recent Advances in Coloproctology

Springer
London
Berlin
Heidelberg
New York
Barcelona
Hong Kong
Milan
Paris
Santa Clara
Singapore
Tokyo

John Beynon and
Nicholas David Carr (Eds)

Recent Advances
in Coloproctology

With 29 Figures

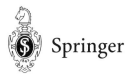
Springer

Mr John Beynon, BSc, MS, FRCS
Mr Nicholas David Carr, MD, FRCS

Department of Colorectal Surgery, Singleton Hospital, Sketty,
Swansea SA2 8QA, UK

Cover illustration: Ch. 5 Fig. 1: Brunel and Kjaer rotating scanner.

ISBN 1-85233-169-0 Springer-Verlag London Berlin Heidelberg

British Library Cataloguing in Publication Data
Recent advances in coloproctology
   1. Colon (Anatomy) – Diseases   2. Rectum – Diseases
   3. Intestines – Diseases
   I. Beynon, John   II. Carr, Nicholas David
616.3′4
ISBN 1852331690

Library of Congress Cataloging-in-Publication Data
Recent advances in coloproctology / [edited by] John Beynon and Nicholas David Carr.
     p.   cm.
   Includes bibliographical references and index.
   ISBN 1-85233-169-0 (alk. paper)
   1. Colon (Anatomy)-Surgery.   2. Rectum–Surgery.   3. Laparoscopic
surgery.   I. Beynon, J. (John)   II. Carr, Nicholas David, 1951–   .
   [DNLM: 1. Colonic Diseases–surgery.   2. Rectal Diseases–surgery.
WI 520 R295 1999]
RD544.R43   1999
617.5′547–dc21
DNLM/DLC   99-24162
for Library of Congress   CIP

Typeset by EXPO Holdings, Malaysia
Printed and bound at the University Press, Cambridge
28/3830-543210 Printed on acid-free paper SPIN 10718621

Preface

Coloproctology has transformed from an uninviting branch of general surgery to a major sub-speciality within its own right. This change has been driven by a number of factors. Anorectal and colonic diseases are common, symptomatically distressing and have, in the past, been managed either inappropriately or unenthusiastically. The marrying of surgical technique with an understanding of the biology of diseases of the colon and anorectum combined with changes in technology and methods of investigation has transformed coloproctology from a purely surgical into a multidisciplinary speciality.

There are many excellent textbooks, which address the subject of coloproctology in a systematic and pragmatic way. Whilst this approach is essential to the orderly teaching of colorectal surgery and related disciplines, times move on and these texts do not necessarily address the current opinion of respected authors who have not only communicated extensively on their subject, but also have an international reputation in their particular field. It is not our intention to compete with authoritative writings, but merely to address certain topics, written by respected authors, which relate to controversial issues within the sub-speciality and which continue to be debated. We feel particularly privileged to have attracted so many experts to have made a contribution to this book.

In these times of 'accelerated' learning, we, the editors, believe this first volume offers an up-to-date synopsis of current thinking on a variety of coloproctological topics and should be of great value to higher surgical trainees and even consultants.

JB & NDC

Contents

List of Contributors

Arthur Allan
Good Hope Hospital
Rectory Road
Sutton Coldfield
West Midlands B75 7RR
UK

David C.C. Bartolo
Royal Infirmary of Edinburgh
Lauriston Place
Edinburgh EH3 9YW
UK

Philip E. Bearn
Good Hope Hospital
Rectory Road
Sutton Coldfield
West Midlands B75 7RR
UK

John Beynon
Singleton Hospital
Sketty
Swansea SA2 8QA
UK

Emin A. Carapeti
Department of Surgery
St Marks Hospital
Northwick Park
Harrow HA1 3UJ
UK

Nicholas D. Carr
Singleton Hospital
Sketty
Swansea SA2 8QA
UK

Timothy A. Cook
Department of Colorectal
    Surgery
John Radcliffe Hospital
Oxford OX1 9DU
UK

Christopher Gatzen
Department of Colorectal
    Surgery
Wycombe Hospital
High Wycombe
Bucks HP11 2TT
UK

Darren M. Gold
Department of Colorectal Surgery
Central Middlesex Hospital NHS
    Trust
Acton Lane, Park Royal
London NW10 7NS
UK

Witold A. Kmiot
St Thomas's Hospital
Lambeth Palace Road
London SE1 7EH
UK

Malcolm G. Lucas
Department of Urological
    Surgery
Morriston Hospital
Swansea SA6 6NL
UK

Neil J. McC. Mortensen
Department of Colorectal
   Surgery
John Radcliffe Hospital
Oxford OX3 9DU
UK

John Nicholls
St Marks Academic Institute
St Marks Hospital
Northwick Park
Harrow HA1 3UJ
UK

Robin K.S. Phillips
Department of Surgery
St Marks Hospital
Northwick Park
Harrow HA1 3UJ
UK

Mara R. Salum
Cleveland Clinic Florida
Department of Colorectal
   Surgery
3000 West Cypress Creek Road
Fort Lauderdale
FL 33309
USA

Giulio A. Santoro
Royal Infirmary of Edinburgh
Lauriston Place
Edinburgh EH3 9YW
UK

Philip F. Schofield
15 St John Street
Manchester M3 4DG
UK

Steven D. Wexner
Cleveland Clinic Florida
Department of Colorectal
   Surgery
3000 West Cypress Creek Road
Fort Lauderdale
FL 33309
USA

1 Complications of Pouch Surgery

R.J. Nicholls and C. Gatzen

Introduction

Restorative proctocolectomy, introduced in the late 1970s, has become the pre-ferred elective operation for the treatment of ulcerative colitis. By the early 1980s, there was considerable experience in many specialist centres and it was apparent that complications were common, often requiring special management. By 1986[1] the incidence of failure had been quantified and defined as the need to remove the pouch and establish a permanent ileostomy. Abscess formation within the pelvis was the most important cause of early failure.

The operation has a low operative mortality of less than 1% even in older patients. Complications are however common, being reported to occur in 20–50% of cases.[1–7]

Failure can be early or late. Initial reports of the operation gave a failure rate of 5–10% in the first year, but it has subsequently become clear that failure continues to occur indefinitely(Fig. 1.1).[8] The chief reasons include sepsis, poor function and ileal mucosal inflammation. Half of all failures over a 10-year period occur in the first year following operation. About 30% of the 5% of patients who develop pelvic sepsis in the post-operative period ultimately fail.

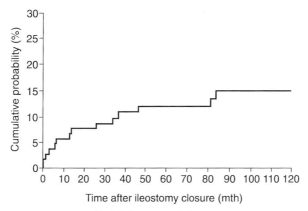

Fig. 1.1. Long-term failure.

Avoidance of Complications

Complications can be minimised by good case selection, an operative technique that pays attention to basic surgical principles of haemostasis, lack of anastomotic tension and the early post-operative recognition of an incipient complication.

Case Selection

Case selection should be based on the pathology of the disease, function of the anal sphincter and the general condition and wishes of the patient.

Pathology

Crohn's Disease

Restorative proctocolectomy has been performed on patients with Crohn's disease. Most of these were erroneously believed to have ulcerative colitis at presentation and were shown to have Crohn's disease on the basis of the subsequent histopathological examination of the resected specimen or the clinical course post-operatively. Failure in patients with Crohn's disease is high, being over 20% in most series, with the notable exception of the report of Panis et al.[9] who found it occurred in only two of 31 patients. However, it is possible that several of these had indeterminate colitis, which has a better prognosis after restorative proctocolectomy than Crohn's disease. Further studies of the results of pouch surgery in Crohn's disease are awaited.

Indeterminate Colitis

This is not a histopathological diagnosis. It is a term given to a small group of patients with inflammatory bowel disease in whom the pathologist cannot distinguish ulcerative colitis from Crohn's disease. Patients may show both macroscopic and microscopic features of each condition in the same specimen. Indeterminate colitis is most often observed in patients having an emergency colectomy for severe acute colitis or toxic megacolon.[10] The severity of inflammation may obscure specific histopathological features, and where the pathologist is unable to deliver a firm diagnosis the clinician should consider clinical and radiological features within the whole framework of the case. Thus, the presence of an anal lesion or any indication of small intestinal inflammation on contrast radiology should be taken to indicate Crohn's disease. Where there is doubt, further biopsies should be taken in any residual large bowel (usually the rectum).

Taking clinical and radiological criteria into account along with the histological features, Wells et al.[11] were able to make a retrospective diagnosis of Crohn's disease or ulcerative colitis in 30 of 46 patients with indeterminate colitis. There were therefore 16 patients in whom the diagnosis remained indeterminate. Of these none developed features of Crohn's disease when followed for a median of 10 years. Thus, a patient with 'indeterminate' colitis without an anal or small intestinal involvement is very unlikely to have Crohn's disease. Pezim et al.[12] reported that patients having indeterminate colitis having had restorative proctocolectomy, fared no worse than patients with unequivocal ulcerative colitis over a 38±18 month period. There is evidence however that over a longer period, patients with indeterminate colitis do have a higher failure rate than those with ulcerative colitis.[13] It is thus essential to establish as far as possible that the patient has ulcerative colitis.

Carcinoma

Patients with a carcinoma of the large bowel are suitable for restorative proctocolectomy under two circumstances. First, there should not be any disseminated disease. Second, the tumour should be amenable to local removal according to accepted principles of cancer clearance. Restorative proctocolectomy is however usually only considered for patients with synchronous carcinomas or carcinomas in the presence of ulcerative colitis or familial adenomatous polyposis.

Severe Acute Colitis

Patients with severe acute colitis, toxic dilatation or perforation should undergo a colectomy with ileostomy and preservation of the rectal stump as a first-stage procedure before embarking on restorative proctectomy. This allows withdrawal of anti-inflammatory medication and the patient to regain general health and self-confidence.

In these circumstances it is desirable to leave a long recto-sigmoid stump to allow the rectum to be found early at a subsequent operation. A short rectal stump may be very difficult to find with the risk of damage to surrounding structures, including the vagina, the seminal vesicles and nerves and vessels on the lateral pelvic wall.

Anal Canal Function

The operation relies on an adequate anal sphincter. It is important therefore to ensure that there is sufficient internal and external sphincter activity and to diagnose a subclinical sphincter tear. Clinical examination, manometry and anal ultrasound should be employed where there is any doubt.

General Factors

Much has been written on whether there should be an age limit. Bauer et al.,[6] reporting a series of 392 patients, found no significant difference in complication rates, frequency of defaecation or incontinence in 326 patients under 50, compared with 66 patients over 50 years. Others are in accord with this observation.[7,14,15] Chronological age should not therefore be a contraindication to the procedure.

It is difficult to refuse a patient on the basis of personality. There are, however, occasional patients who may not be temperamentally suited to the operation given its potential problems. Extensive consultation and counselling is essential for all patients. A specialist pouch support nurse can be very helpful in this respect. Patients should never be pressurised to have the operation and should be given every opportunity to have access to the clinician and to patient support groups of which there are now many.

Operative Technique

Avoidance of Ileoanal Anastomotic Breakdown

The most important complication is that of breakdown of the ileoanal anastomosis with pelvic abscess formation. As with any other anastomosis, tension, ischaemia and contamination are the three most important factors leading to this.

Tension

The mesenteric vessels tend to restrain the terminal ileum as it is drawn down to the anal level and may cause tension on the anastomosis. This may lead to dehiscence at one point leading to pelvic sepsis, or there may be complete retraction resulting in subsequent stricture formation.

Care should therefore be taken to achieve adequate mobility. The ileocolic artery and vein are not necessary for perfusion of the terminal ileum and should be divided. The mesentery should be mobilised up to the duodenum and any intrinsic adhesions within it carefully divided. A trial descent is very valuable to assess tension. Where a manual ileoanal anastomosis is intended, the bowel is divided at the anorectal junction leaving an open anal stump. A stay suture is placed on the antimesenteric border of the ileum which will form the ileal component of the anastomosis. This is then drawn through the anus by an operator stationed at the perineum. If the ileum is adequately mobile to descend to the dentate line, it will do so after reconstruction of the reservoir. If it does not reach at this stage further mobilisation of the mesentery will be necessary. It might be necessary to divide a particular vessel within the mesentery deemed to be creating tension. This must be done with great care, ensuring that perfusion of the terminal ileum is adequate after division. Application of a bulldog clamp to the selected vessel before division will enable this to be determined by the presence or absence of submucosal arterial bleeding from the divided end of the ileum.

While there is no difference in pelvic sepsis rates after stapled or hand-sutured ileoanal anastomosis in randomised trials,[16,17] the former has the advantage that the anastomosis is placed at the anal rectal junction lying at about 2 cm above the dentate line. In cases with a short mesentery, where adequate mobility is questionable, a stapled anastomosis will result in less tension and should therefore be carried out.

When a defunctioning ileostomy is used, the surgeon should make sure that this does not increase tension on blood vessels within the mesentery. If it does, the potential value of an ileostomy is outweighed by the risk of the tension causing ischaemia.

Haemostasis

It is difficult to achieve complete haemostasis in the pelvis after rectal removal. There are however particular sites of bleeding that the surgeon should be aware of. These include the divided anal stump if a manual anastomosis is to be carried out, the branches of the internal iliac artery entering the lower rectum and any vessel within the mesorectum if a perimuscular dissection has been carried out. The anatomical argument over the presence or absence of the middle rectal vessels is not relevant since blood vessels enter the lower rectum laterally on each side in all cases whether from middle rectal vessels or another branch of the internal iliac artery.

Factors Influencing Future Function

Pouch Design

There is an inverse relationship between capacitance of the reservoir and frequency of defecation. This is true for ileal or colonic pouches.[18,19] The pouch should therefore be of adequate size. If a J two-loop pouch is to be used, there is agreement that each limb should be about 20 cm long. This construction may actually increase tension on the ileoanal anastomosis since the most mobile part of the terminal ileum is located about 15 cm proximal to the ileocaecal valve. Three-loop (S) and four-loop (W) designs and the Kock-configuration design[20] have a higher starting volume, and long-term follow-up indicates that frequency and its variance are less with these constructions.[8] Size of reservoir is one of the few factors influencing function over which the surgeon has control.

The distal ileal segment of the three-loop (S) pouch results in impedance to defaecation.[21] For this reason it has been superseded by designs that allow the reservoir to be directly anastomosed to the anal stump.

Anal Sphincter Damage

The anal sphincter can be damaged by both stapled and manual ileoanal anastomoses. Resting anal tone post-operatively is reduced after almost all manual, and in about 50% of stapled, anastomoses.[16] In performing a manual endoanal anastomosis of the anus, dilatation by the anal retractor should be kept to a minimum. The surgeon should think constantly of the effect that dilation will have upon sphincter tone.

Ileoanal Anastomosis

The level of the ileoanal anastomosis has an influence on the subsequent course. It should be placed at the anorectal junction or more distally. An anastomosis of ileal pouch to the distal rectum may have three adverse consequences. First, inflamed mucosa is left behind and this may be symptomatic, causing discomfort, bleeding and a frequent desire to defaecate. This condition has been given the name of "strip proctitis".[22] Second, it seems that emptying of the reservoir is impeded if part of the rectum is retained. This causes the frequent passage of small volumes of stool. Third, the residual rectal mucosa is still at risk of developing carcinoma in the long term.

It is easier to control the level of the ileoanal anastomosis using a manual endoanal technique combined with a mucosectomy. If a stapled technique is to be used, great care is necessary to apply the transverse stapler sufficiently distal to avoid leaving any rectum.

Pelvic Nerve Damage

Perimuscular dissection of the rectum as described by Lee and Dowling[23] avoids any damage to the pelvic nerves which might lead to urinary and sexual dysfunction.[24] This technique is not routinely practised since it is time-consuming but it allows confident reassurance to the patient that nerve function will be preserved. Keeping close to the rectum requires the division of branches of the superior rectal artery within the mesorectum as they enter the rectal wall. In patients with dysplasia or carcinoma, however, the rectal dissection should be carried out in the anatomical plane between mesorectum and the presacral tissues in accordance with the principles of cancer surgery.

Normal Post-operative Course

In-patient

During the first 24 hours satisfactory progress will be indicated by stable vital signs and adequate urine output. If a pelvic drain has been inserted, it should be removed the next morning. Drainage is usually about 200 ml during the first 12 hours post-operatively. The ileostomy begins to function within 2–5 days. Water and electrolyte (chiefly sodium) balance may require special attention if ileostomy output is high, which it often is at this stage. Sodium depletion is common and its possibility should be explained to the patient. Oral electrolyte mixture may be required and the patient should be encouraged to add salt to food, as solid diet is reintroduced. The electrolyte mixture contains sodium in a concentration of 60 mmol per litre. This is about half the sodium concentration in ileostomy effluent. The patient must know therefore that relying on the electrolyte mixture alone is not adequate.

During the post-operative period, almost all patients experience a discharge of altered bloody mucus through the anus. This is normal and the patient can be reassured that it will settle. However, the passage of fresh blood is a different matter and usually indicates a secondary infection associated with ileoanal breakdown.

If all goes well post-operatively, there is no need to perform a digital examination of the anastomosis. Where breakdown is clinically suspected it should be performed. The finger should easily enter the pouch allowing palpation of the anastomosis. Mobility and lack of induration indicate satisfactory healing. If there is evidence of a defect, nothing further should be done at this stage provided the patient is clinically well. Where there is evidence of a larger defect associated with abscess formation, an examination under anaesthetic with drainage of the collection should be performed. The patient will be instructed in stoma care, where an ileostomy is present. The usual duration of in-patient stay is 8–10 days.

Out-patient

The patient should be seen at about a month after leaving hospital. An assessment of recovery will be made, with particular attention to any evidence of sodium depletion. A digital examination of the anastomosis is performed.

In some patients, the anastomosis feels stenosed. This may be due to a true stenosis or more commonly may simply be due to adhesions across the anastomosis which will yield to gentle pressure with the finger. A contrast radiograph of the pouch (pouchogram) should be carried out if satisfactory anastomotic healing is in doubt. If a small track is shown, the examination should be repeated after a month or so. In the absence of any sign of anastomotic defect or pelvic sepsis, it will be possible to close the ileostomy (Fig. 1.2). The patient should be warned

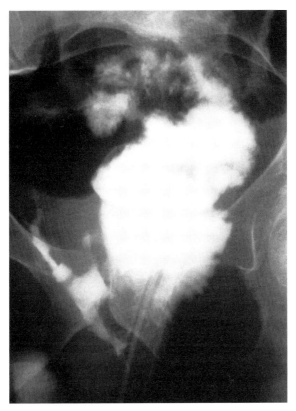

Fig. 1.2. Leak from pouch-anal anastomosis.

that following closure function may be disturbed for several weeks but initial high frequency and episodes of leakage are likely to improve with time. Anti-diarrhoeal medication should be given when frequency is troublesome. In the early post-operative period, barrier cream should be applied to the perianal skin as a routine to prevent excoriation.

Early Postoperative Complications

Fever

Fever in the post-operative period is most likely to be due to abdominal or pelvic sepsis. Other causes of infection in the chest, urinary tract and wound should be excluded. Examination of the abdomen may reveal clinical evidence of indura-tion or tenderness. Ultrasound examination may confirm the presence of an abdominal collection.

Pelvic sepsis

The diagnosis of pelvic sepsis is less straightforward, since it can be present despite an apparently normal digital examination of the anastomotic area. Ultrasound for pelvic sepsis is unreliable, as the pouch itself confuses the ultra-sonographic picture. If digital examination is not diagnostic, then a computed tomography (CT) scan should be considered. If there is clinical suspicion of sepsis, an examination under anaesthetic with drainage of any abscess should be performed. This should also be carried out if the patient has passed fresh blood per anum, giving warning of secondary haemorrhage that may be associated with sepsis. Occasionally, fever may be due to retained infected mucus within the pouch and will settle on drainage via a proctoscope.

Haemorrhage

Bleeding occurring within the first few hours of surgery may be intraperitoneal or within the lumen of the reservoir. It is likely to stop in most cases, but clearly where it does not, re-exploration is needed. Where the clinical picture suggests that a significant intraperitoneal haemorrhage has occurred, exploration should be recommended even if there is no compromise to the circulation. Early re-operation with evacuation of clot will remove a potential source of morbidity, since an infected haematoma may develop into a serious situation leading to pelvic sepsis and compromise of the operation.

If laparotomy is required, access to the bleeding may be impossible owing to the presence of the pouch, if this is coming from low within the pelvis, for example from the lateral pelvic wall or the anal stump. Under this circumstance it may be necessary to detach the ileoanal anastomosis, secure the bleeding and then re-anastomose. While this may seem a major undertaking, it is little different from the initial pouch operation and will give the patient the best chance of avoiding a haematoma-related complication. If the bleeding cannot be arrested, the pelvis should be packed and the pouch exteriorised as a mucous fistula with the hope of a future re-anastomosis.

Bleeding into the reservoir or at the ileoanal anastomosis will require an examination under anaesthetic with irrigation of the reservoir to obtain vision. There is a good prospect of identifying a bleeding vessel and arresting it either by coagulation or by under-running it with a suture.

Secondary haemorrhage is associated with sepsis. When intraluminal, the patient will discharge fresh blood per anum. The patient should undergo an examination under anaesthetic forthwith and the site of bleeding and any concurrent sepsis dealt with. Rarely, secondary haemorrhage occurs within the abdomen, and laparotomy may be necessary. If haemorrhage is due to general oozing within an infected cavity, this should be packed with or without detachment of the reservoir from the anal canal.

Pelvic sepsis is the most common cause of early failure. The reported incidence varies considerably with rates ranging from 5% to over 30%.[1] To some extent this may be due to different interpretations of the definition by surgeons reporting their results. The term pelvic sepsis is used to describe a serious septic event requiring drainage by the abdominal route. Others have used the term to include any case in which there is an anastomotic complication however trivial. It is difficult from publications to determine the criteria used to record this complication. It is probable that pelvic sepsis resulting in the need for drainage occurs in about 5–10% of cases in most series.

Surgical factors that might influence a subsequent anastomotic breakdown have been discussed above. There has been much argument on the relative merits of manual versus stapled anastomosis. In randomised trials, however, no significant difference has been shown for anastomotic morbidity or function after either method of anastomosis.[16,17] The surgeon should be competent in both techniques, since there are times where one may be preferable over the other, despite the surgeon's routine practice.

Pelvic sepsis is a strong indicator of subsequent failure. Of a consecutive series of 340 cases, 42 developed an anastomotic complication based on stringent criteria. Of these, 14 (33%) required removal of the reservoir and the establishment of a permanent ileostomy (personal observations), giving an overall failure rate due to sepsis of 4%.

Ischaemia

Ischaemia is uncommon, but is a serious event. Poor perfusion of the reservoir may result from injudicious division of mesenteric vessels in trying to achieve mobility, stretching on the mesenteric vessels owing to tension or to postoperative hypotension, resulting in poor gut perfusion.

The patient develops toxaemia with raised pulse and white cell count. The ischaemia process may lead to complete necrosis of the pouch or to an ischaemic ileitis predominantly affecting the mucosa.

The condition should be suspected if there is deterioration of the patient's condition with the passage of copious bloodstained secretion per anum. An early endoscopy should be carried out using a conventional rigid sigmoidoscope with suction available. The mucosa may be obviously necrotic or it may show evidence of oedema and ulceration with haemorrhage. In the former circumstance, urgent re-operation is required with removal of the necrotic segment and the establishment of an ileostomy. Where there is an ileitis, it may be reasonable to treat the patient expectantly in the hope that the condition will resolve. If it does so the patient may however be left with a small contracted reservoir.

Intestinal Obstruction

Small bowel obstruction in the post-operative period is reported to occur in 5–25% cases.[1,5] Obstruction may be due to early adhesion formation or to a mechanical complication of the ileostomy. In the latter circumstance, lateral space obstruction with herniation of the small bowel around the stoma can occur. The ileostomy may also rotate[25] leading to intermittent obstruction. More commonly however, obstruction is due to a narrow trephine.

Adhesion formation may result in a localised band or bands causing occlusion at a definite point. More often however, the process may result in loops of bowel being matted together by diffuse inflammatory adhesions.

A bio-reabsorbable membrane of chemically modified hyaluronic acid and carboxymethylcellulose (Seprafilm) and a liquid preparation of sodium hyaluronate (Sepracote) have been recently developed and are presently being assessed, based on two reports of a randomised controlled blinded prospective multicentre trial.[26,27] These report that the membrane when placed under the abdominal wound during restorative proctocolectomy with diverting ileostomy decreases the rate of adhesion formation by nearly 50% when assessed at the time of ileostomy closure. Further work is in progress, but if such material significantly reduces adhesion formation with a reduction in clinical obstruction this would be a significant advance.

In patients having a one-stage procedure or in those in whom a temporary ileostomy has been closed, obstruction may be due to hold-up at the pouch-anal level. It is essential to exclude this possibility by the passage of a sigmoidoscope into the reservoir, which will result in the escape of intestinal contents and relief of the obstruction.

Obstruction may follow closure of the ileostomy. This may be due to an inadequate lumen, but sometimes the level is located more proximally. The explanation for this is not clear, since the ileostomy had been working satisfactorily before closure.

Management of obstruction should be conservative wherever possible. Strangulation is uncommon, but any evidence of worsening pain, abdominal tenderness and leucocytosis should prompt early intervention. In most cases it will be possible to wait, sometimes with intravenous nutritional support.

Subsequently, chronic obstruction or intermittent obstructive episodes can occur. A decision whether to intervene or not is essentially a clinical one, but this may be helped by water-soluble contrast small bowel radiology. This may identify the site of obstruction and if the condition does not improve spontaneously or if obstructive episodes persist at an unacceptable frequency, then surgery will be necessary. Chronic obstruction is a cause of poor function, especially frequency of defecation.

Ileostomy

The use of a temporary ileostomy was recommended in the early days of restorative proctocolectomy. Most surgeons still adopt it as a routine, since it is felt that the consequences of an anastomotic breakdown causing sepsis are mitigated. It is, however, a significant source of morbidity. A quarter of all complications were due to the stoma in a series of patients with familial adenomatous polyposis undergoing restorative proctocolectomy.[28] Thow[29] described a technique involving intubation of the small intestine that avoided the need for an ileostomy, but there was a significant incidence of late sepsis. However, it is impossible to know whether this would not have occurred had an ileostomy been carried out. Everett[30] reported 60 patients, of whom 20 had no ileostomy. Four (20%) developed a significant complication, but only two of these required a subsequent stoma, giving an overall stoma rate of 10%. Hospital stay was significantly shorter compared with the two-stage procedure with a mean of 11.7 days versus 27.9 days respectively. The authors recommended a selective policy, in which an ileostomy could be avoided in the absence of risk factors for an anastomotic breakdown, including good general condition of the patient, a tension-free well-perfused anastomosis and satisfactory haemostasis.

Grobler et al.[31] found no difference in the incidence of pelvic sepsis in a randomised trial comparing 22 patients with no ileostomy with 23 in whom this was carried out. In both of these groups only one case of pelvic sepsis occurred. This trial adopted a selective approach to entry whereby patients considered to have significant risk factors for pelvic sepsis were not entered. Nevertheless, the data indicate that a one-stage procedure correctly selected does not appear to increase the risk for the patient.

If the strategy of a one-stage procedure is adopted, the surgeon must be prepared to carry out an ileostomy in the early post-operative period in the event of sepsis occurring. The incidence of this being necessary is about 10–20%. Thus the surgeon has to balance the disadvantage of re-operation in a few cases against the advantage of shorter post-operative hospitalisation in the majority as well as the incidence of complications due to the stoma itself.

Loop ileostomy carries a significant morbidity. It may not achieve the intended purpose of complete faecal diversion, and inadequate defunctioning was thought to be related to an increased incidence of pelvic sepsis. Reported rates of ileostomy creation range from 5.7%[32] to 41%[33], although in this last series only two patients required hospital admission.

Most important complications of ileostomy formation include excessive water and electrolyte loss, retraction and intestinal obstruction, which requires laparotomy in 4–6% of cases.[32,33]

Closure results in fistula formation with or without peritonitis in 2–19%. The procedure should be performed with great care by an experienced operator. Difficulties can be encountered where there are dense adhesions around the stoma. These are likely to resolve and it is wise to allow an interval of 8 weeks or more following the original restorative proctocolectomy before closing the stoma. If difficulties are encountered, the abdomen should be opened to obtain adequate access to allow safe mobilisation. The patient should be warned of this eventuality beforehand.

At least 50 cm of small intestine will lie distal to the loop ileostomy. These include about 40 cm forming the reservoir and a further 10–20 cm between the pouch and the ileostomy itself. This results in a higher output than would occur from an end ileostomy placed in the terminal ileum. Volumes may exceed three or more litres per 24 hours and can rapidly lead to sodium and water depletion with features of weakness, postural hypertension, nausea and anorexia creating a vicious circle with further diminution of oral salt and water intake. The treatment is sodium and water repletion by intravenous normal saline and once oral intake has been resumed, the patient must take an adequate amount of salt in the diet. It may be necessary to supplement this by an electrolyte solution as indicated above. There is a natural tendency for a high initial output to diminish over the first few days to weeks post-operatively, but if it persists, early closure of the ileostomy is indicated, provided the ileoanal anastomosis is satisfactory.

Late Post-operative Complications

Delayed Sepsis

Delayed sepsis can manifest clinically in two ways. An abscess cavity with track formation into the intestinal lumen may persist, or a fistula may suddenly appear as an unheralded occurrence.

In the former case, drainage under general anaesthetic has a reasonable prospect of healing the fistula. Failure despite this measure may necessitate removal of the pouch or an attempted salvage procedure. Salvage is likely to require abdominal surgery. In the case of a fistula from the ileoanal anastomosis, this may require detachment of the pouch from the anal canal and its exteriorisation as a mucous fistula on the anterior abdominal wall. It is then hoped that with time the sepsis will heal, allowing re-anastomosis again through an abdominal approach. Major salvage of this type is no mean undertaking and very careful discussion with the patient concerning the options is essential. The surgeon has a responsibility to make it clear that the chances of salvage in this situation are not high. Armed with these facts, the patient should be allowed to decide, bearing in mind the further hospitalisation, risk of complications and low prospect of success that a salvage procedure for sepsis involves.

Fistulation from the reservoir itself may close spontaneously following drainage of any associated abscess. If it does not, then surgical closure will be necessary. The success of such a procedure will depend upon the level of the fistula. If it is located in the upper part of the pouch, access via an abdominal incision should be straightforward, with a high prospect of successful closure. If on the other hand the origin is from a fistula from the lower part of the pouch, it may be impossible to obtain access without taking down the ileoanal anastomosis, as described above. If this is necessary, the surgeon must make a decision whether to revise the anastomosis with drainage of the chronic abscess cavity or whether to excise the pouch or to exteriorise it as a mucous fistula. These options should be discussed fully with the patient pre-operatively.

Ozuner et al.[34] have reported a series of 59 patients with fistulation. An overall success rate of 60% was obtained following surgical closure. In the group of patients with fistulation in the lower part of the pouch, the success rate was less than 50%, while in contrast it was over 80% where the fistula was high.

Pouch-Vaginal and Pouch-Perineal Fistula

Fistulae of these types are extrasphincteric. They result in faecal incontinence and in almost all patients surgical treatment is obligatory.

The condition was first reported by Wong et al.[35] in 1985. The pouch-perineal fistula is the male equivalent of pouch-vaginal fistula. In a review of 304 patients operated on in 11 centres, 21 (6.4%) patients developed pouch-vaginal fistulae.[36] The reported incidence in the literature in general ranges from 2% to 17%.[37,38] The condition does not appear to be disease-related and only rarely is Crohn's disease identified in a patient with pouch-vaginal fistula. However, there is a history of pelvic sepsis or anastomotic complication in the immediate post-operative period in over 60% of patients with pouch-vaginal fistula.[39] Intra-operative vaginal injury and subsequent pouchitis appear also to be aetiological factors. The type of pouch used does not correlate with the occurrence of this complication, but there is some evidence to indicate that it is more common after a stapled than a manual anastomosis.

Pouch-vaginal fistula can occur in the early post-operative period before closure of the ileostomy or following closure. The interval between closure of the ileostomy and fistula development can be many years, though the median interval was 8 months in a series of 21 cases.[39]

Pouch-vaginal fistula results in leakage of flatus or faeces per vaginam. Flatus alone may not necessarily indicate fistula formation and careful examination is essential. There is usually a point of induration palpable on the posterior vaginal wall and palpation of the ileoanal anastomosis per anum may reveal an obvious opening, but this is not evident in all cases. Gentle insufflation of air through a sigmoidoscope into the pouch may be followed by bubbles emerging through the

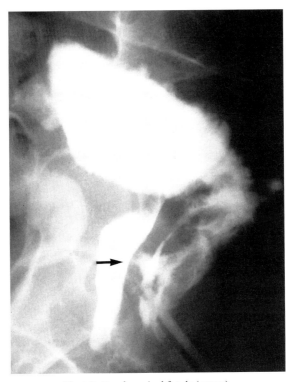

Fig. 1.3. Pouch-vaginal fistula (*arrow*).

posterior vaginal wall, best visualised with a proctoscope placed in the vagina. A water-soluble contrast X-ray should be carried out, but examination under anaesthetic is the best method of diagnosis when this is in doubt (Fig. 1.3).

Treatment is difficult. Simple laying open is obviously not possible and surgical closure may fail. Where the fistula is very small with an intermittent discharge of flatus only, it may be wise simply to observe the patient. Where the symptom is significant, however, surgical closure should be attempted. A defunctioning ileostomy should be carried out in all cases. In many this will be necessary to relieve the incontinence, but it will also give surgical closure the best chance of success.

Simple drainage or defunctioning alone is very unlikely to result in healing without an attempt at surgical closure. Fleshman et al.[40] reported this to occur in only one of 16 patients treated in this way initially, although Groom et al.[39] reported spontaneous closure in four of six fistulae developing before closure of the ileostomy, in contrast to none of 15 patients where the complication developed after closure.

Numerous techniques for closure have been tried, including fistulotomy followed by sphincter repair, pouch advancement flap, detachment of the ileoanal anastomosis and direct transvaginal closure.

Distal advancement of the ileoanal anastomosis is the procedure of choice where the fistula arises from a stapled anastomosis. The level of this will be more proximal than if a manual anastomosis had been carried out and there is therefore some room for manoeuvre distally by bringing the anastomosis down to the level of the dentate line. However, such a procedure will involve an abdominal approach to mobilise the pouch and detach the ileoanal anastomosis. The new anastomosis will need to be carried out manually. Using this technique in this selected group of patients, the authors has succeeded in five out of five cases.

Where the fistula lies at a lower level, as occurs following an original manual anastomosis, advancement of the anastomosis is not possible. In this situation local techniques should be employed. An endoanal pouch advancement flap was reported to result in success in six of nine patients.[40] Others have had a similar experience.[5]

A direct approach through the posterior vaginal wall has the advantage of avoiding damage to the anal sphincter that can occur using an endoanal approach. The vaginal opening is circumcised and the fistula track dissected to its entry into the gut tube. The resulting defect is directly sutured and the vagina closed over the repair. Using this technique, six of eight cases were successfully closed (personal observations) and similar results have been obtained by others.[41] Where the internal opening lies within the anal canal, access using a transvaginal approach may be impossible owing to the presence of the anal sphincter. This can be overcome by division of the sphincter to allow direct repair of the anal canal epithelium followed by repair of the sphincter.

While Crohn's disease is rarely a cause in most series, Lee et al.[42] reported 25 patients, of whom 12 were subsequently reclassified as having Crohn's disease. Twenty patients underwent a transanal repair (advancement flap 12, direct repair 6, neo-ileal anastomosis 2). Of those without Crohn's disease having transanal repair, 10 healed, one lost the pouch and one had a recurrence. Of the 12 patients with Crohn's disease, the prognosis was poor, with six requiring excision of the pouch and only three experiencing healing.

Fistulation from the ileoanal anastomosis to the perineum is the male equivalent of a pouch-vaginal fistula. Some of these cases may be managed satisfactorily by the insertion of a Seton suture to offer drainage. Surprisingly, there may be only a small amount of new muco-purulent secretion and the patient may be content to accept this as a reasonable price to pay for retaining the reservoir.

Anal Pain and Ulceration

Anal pain is common in the post-operative period. The anastomosis will produce some discomfort in almost all cases, but if severe or persisting, an additional lesion should be suspected. The causes of pain include a peri-anastomotic collection, anal canal ulceration, anal fissure, and inflammation of a detached part of the anoderm as a result of a partial ileoanal breakdown.

An examination under anaesthetic will enable a diagnosis to be made and appropriate action taken. An abscess should be drained. Ulceration and fissure formation should be treated conservatively with application of local steroids and barrier cream, and also glyceryl trinitrate (GTN) ointment in the case of fissure. Pain may resolve on direct steroid injection as described by Hughes et al.[43]

Where there is no ileostomy, anti-diarrhoeals should be given to reduce frequency. Occasionally in this situation ulceration is so extensive and painful that re-establishment of the ileostomy may be necessary. Before resorting to this it is worth trying a period of endoluminal defunctioning by placing a large-bore retention catheter in the pouch for a few days. Drainage via the catheter is often surprisingly good and the anoderm no longer in contact with faeces is given an opportunity to heal.

Sometimes the severity and indolence of anal ulceration raises the possibility of Crohn's disease. A review of available histopathological material should be made and new biopsies taken from the reservoir, and contrast radiology of the small intestine performed. Usually no conclusive evidence of Crohn's disease is found, and in some patients the anal disease resolves spontaneously.

Anastomotic Stricture

Stricture of the ileoanal anastomosis is usually due to a dehiscence. Where this is partial and results in the occurrence of a pelvic abscess, extramural fibrosis is responsible. Where there is a retraction of the ileal reservoir from the anal stump, a cylinder of denuded tissue results. Even when abscess formation does not occur, a stricture will develop owing to healing by secondary intention with fibrosis. Ischaemia of the ileal reservoir immediately above the anastomosis will also result in a stricture.

The overall incidence of this complication varies considerably, but the pooled experience of several units reported an instance of 20–30%.[1] There is evidence that the complication is more common after a stapled than a hand-sutured anastomosis (Fig. 1.4). In a retrospective study, Senapati reported respective rates of 17% and 42%.[44]

Most strictures can be managed by dilatation. Usually this is necessary on one occasion only, but in a small minority surgical revision may be necessary. The

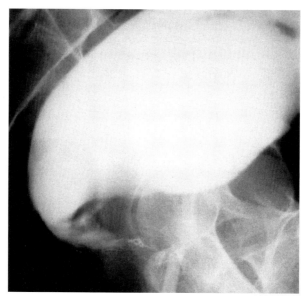

Fig. 1.4. Stenosis of the ileoanal reservoir.

response to dilatation will depend upon the length and tightness of the stricture. A long stricture due to retraction or ischaemia is likely to require surgical revision. Recurrent stenosis after dilatation may be due to persisting pelvic sepsis and imaging may be indicated to identify this.

Dysfunction

Poor function is a major cause of late failure. It is usually manifest by frequency.

Frequency

The average frequency of defaecation after restorative proctocolectomy ranges from four to six times per 24 hours. However, there is a wide variance around this mean, which is skewed, with more patients having a frequency of seven or more times than of three or less. About 20–50% of patients experience a night evacuation of one or more times per week. There is normally a gradual decrease in frequency following closure of the ileostomy over subsequent weeks up to 18 months. Frequency varies according to diet and timing of meals and patients often learn how to optimise their frequency.

Patients with troublesome night-time frequency should be advised to have the evening meal early and to defaecate just before going to bed. The liberal use of anti-diarrhoeal agents, including loperamide, codeine phosphate and Lomotil should be advised. Patients can adjust the timing of these to give optimal reduction of frequency. Some patients are able to identify certain foods that evoke fre-

Table 1.1 Causes of frequency

1. Mechanical
   Distal segment
   Stenosis
   Retained rectal stump

2. Functional
   Chronic pelvic sepsis
   Chronic intestinal obstruction
   Disturbed physiology
      Sphincter weakness
      Small capacitance
      Excessive stool volume
      Intestinal bacterial growth
      Motility disorder

3. Pouchitis

4. Crohn's disease

quency. Advice from a dietician or pouch support nurse can be very useful in this respect. In the early adaptive phase, patients should be encouraged that frequency will diminish with time.

Causes of Frequency

There are many causes for frequency (Table 1.1), pouchitis being only one. It is essential therefore to assess the patient fully, by a careful history and anorectal examination supplemented by special investigations including histopathology, radiology and physiology.

History and Examination

From the history it will be possible to identify patients who experience the frequent passage of small volumes of stool, indicating incomplete emptying of the pouch, which suggests an evacuation disorder. Patients with urgency may have an incompetent anal sphincter. Those with pouchitis usually pass large volumes of watery stool, and may in addition experience abdominal cramps and malaise with the occasional appearance of an activity-related extra-alimentary manifestation. History and examination may also identify patients with chronic intestinal obstruction and chronic pelvic sepsis.

Outflow mechanical obstruction will be evident on physical examination. This is manifest by stenosis, a long distal ileal segment and the increasingly observed complication of pouch-rectal anastomosis. Stenosis is evident on digital examination, which will enable an assessment of severity judged by the diameter of the anastomosis and the degree of surrounding induration. A distal ileal segment is now rarely seen as very few S reservoirs are being constructed. Digital examination and rigid sigmoidoscopy will demonstrate the ileoanal anastomosis and also the exit of the reservoir, placed several centimetres more proximal. A pouch-rectal anastomosis is recognised on palpation lying a variable distance above the puborectalis sling. Rigid sigmoidoscopy will show inflamed rectal mucosa below with the contrasting appearance of ileal mucosa above. Biopsies at each level should be taken.

Investigations

Plain radiography of the abdomen may show dilated loops indicating obstruction. Contrast radiology of the small bowel may identify its site. A contrast enema (pouchogram) will show the presence of a mechanical obstruction by demonstrating dilatation of the pouch with narrowing distally. It will also identify a retained rectal stump, a small capacitance reservoir and a contracted reservoir due to inflammation. Videopouchography may be useful to assess the dynamic behaviour of the pouch, particularly with regard to emptying. Physiological assessment of the anal sphincter will detect a functional weakness of both internal and external sphincter and anal ultrasound may identify an occult mechanical sphincter injury, for example due to subclinical obstetric damage. Volumetry and compliance studies will confirm a small capacitance reservoir, with some indication whether it has become contracted by disease.

Mechanical Outflow Obstruction

Mechanical outflow obstruction to the pouch results in poor emptying with the frequent passage of small volumes of stool. There are three main causes for this:

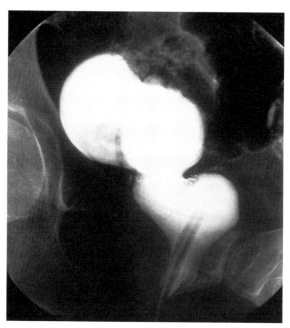

Fig. 1.5. Pouch-rectal anastomosis.

ileoanal stenosis, a retained rectal stump following a pouch-rectal anastomosis and the presence of a distal ileal segment in patients having a three-loop (S) reconstruction (Fig. 1.5).

The diagnosis of incomplete evacuation is suspected by the history and confirmed by anorectal examination. Dilatation of the pouch above an obstructing outlet lesion may be obvious. Residual volume after defaecation can usually be demonstrated by the passage of a catheter into the reservoir. In patients with a retained rectal stump, the anastomosis (almost always stapled) is palpable at a variable distance above the anorectal junction. The rectal mucosa distal to this level can be seen on proctoscopy, and biopsy from this area will show features typical of ulcerative colitis in almost all patients. A pouchogram will show a dilated reservoir and the outlet abnormality and effectiveness of emptying can be gauged on a post-evacuation film. Videopouchography may be a more useful guide to assessing evacuation.

Management of these patients is likely to require major revisional surgery. The aim is to remove the cause of obstruction, with formation of an anastomosis directly between the pouch and the mid-anal canal. The operation should be covered by a temporary ileostomy.

The indication for such salvage surgery must depend upon the perceived chance of success weighed against the prospect of complications and further ultimate disappointment. Much will depend upon the desires of the patient. The results of such surgery are now beginning to appear.[45-47] In a series of 16 patients, including nine with a long efferent limb and six with a stricture, two had a major complication.[48] Fifteen patients had the ileostomy closed and in these, frequency of defaecation fell from a median value of 15 to 6 times per 24 hours. Of 10 incontinent patients, five became continent and four were improved.[46] In a recent analysis of 17 patients undergoing revisional surgery for a retained rectal stump with pouch-rectal anastomosis, a major complication occurred in one and the reservoir was removed in three cases. In the 12 patients available for assessment of function, median frequency fell from 14 to 7 times per 24 hours, with urgency improved in most patients. Prevention is better than cure and the importance of avoiding a pouch-rectal anastomosis cannot be over-emphasised.

Functional

Some patients suffer from poor evacuation in the absence of any mechanical outflow abnormality. Pouchography usually shows a dilated pouch with poor emptying. There may be inadequate force of contraction of the reservoir, which gets progressively worse as it becomes dilated, and some degree of failure of relaxation of the pelvic floor. Some of these patients may show evidence of paradoxical puborectalis contraction.[49] Treatment is difficult, since the nature of the disturbance is unknown. Catheterisation of the reservoir often produces relief. This often seems to be required indefinitely, but occasionally it can be dispensed with after several weeks to months. Perhaps in this circumstance, muscle tone of the reservoir has been allowed to recover following relief of over-distension. It may be that biofeedback has a role in treating this condition.[49]

Chronic Pelvic Sepsis

This represents the end stage of an acute anastomotic complication. Chronic pelvic sepsis may be associated with poor function owing to the local rigidity of the tissues and possibly by irritation of the ileal reservoir. If drainage has already failed, major abdominal surgery is unlikely to result in its resolution. If this is the case, excision of the reservoir with the establishment of a permanent ileostomy should be recommended. If on the other hand there is an abscess that the surgeon feels is practicable to drain, this should be carried out.

Sphincter Weakness

Damage to the anal sphincter may occur during construction of the ileoanal anastomosis. This is more likely to happen after a manual than a stapled technique. Obstetric injury may have occurred. The combination of urgency with frequency should alert suspicion that a weak sphincter is the cause of the dysfunction. Anal ultrasound should demonstrate a sphincter laceration where present and if so, repair should be advised. Diffuse weakness of the anal sphincter is more difficult to treat. In a group of 11 patients undergoing sphincter repair for diffuse weakness or lacerated injury, only four ultimately avoided a permanent ileostomy (Engel, Nicholls, unpublished observations). The prognosis in this group would appear therefore to be poor. Perhaps more recent developments in continence surgery, including dynamic graciloplasty or implantation of the artificial bowel sphincter may have a place. There is as yet little information on the outcome when these are applied to patients with incontinence after pouch surgery.

Passive incontinence is not infrequent and may occur particularly at night. This is largely due to low internal sphincter tone. There is some evidence that the application of phenylephrene ointment to the perianal skin may help these patients by improving internal sphincter function and raising anal canal pressure (Carapeti et al., unpublished observation).

Small Capacitance Reservoir

The original ileoanal procedure described by Ravitch and Sabiston[50] used a straight segment of terminal ileum for the neorectum. While some of these patients had satisfactory function, the majority experienced frequency and urgency clearly due to inadequate capacitance. Heppel et al.[51] showed that capacitance was indirectly related to frequency. This was subsequently shown for the ileal reservoir.[18] Balloon volumetry will identify such cases. This measures the threshold for sensation and for urgency as well as the maximal tolerable volume (MTV). There is a wide variance of the volumes, but an MTV of less than 200 ml is likely to be significant. Salvage is possible in this group, but will involve an abdominal revision of the reservoir with its replacement or augmentation.

Pouchitis

The diagnosis of pouchitis requires histological evidence of acute inflammation within the reservoir and this must be in association with the presence of clinical symptoms of the condition and endoscopic evidence of inflammation. Many of these patients will respond to antibacterial treatment. Such a response does not necessarily make the diagnosis of pouchitis, however. There is a group of patients without histological inflammation in the pouch who also respond to antibacterial treatment. These may have intestinal bacterial overgrowth, but at the present time this is not proven. It is likely, however, that further study will confirm the existence of this condition.

Symptomatic inflammation of the pouch will develop in up to 7–40% of patients who undergo this surgery. Patients present with crampy abdominal pain, fever, rectal bleeding and diarrhoea, and they may have either acute intermittent attacks or a chronic pouchitis syndrome. Most reported cases of pouchitis have occurred in patients with a previous history of ulcerative colitis, whereas complications develop in only a handful of patients with familial adenomatous polyposis (FAP).

Aetiology

Pouchitis is probably a multifactorial condition involving genetic, immune, microbial and toxic mediators. No clear microbiological factor has yet been shown to play a part in the aetiology, but the marked increase in the anaerobe/aerobe ratio in pouches to 100 : 1, compared with 4 : 1 in ileostomy effluent is noteworthy. The evidence to date indicates that it shares some of the cellular and cytokine features that characterise infective colitis. Setti Carraro et al.[52] and Apel et al.[53] showed that villous atrophy, and acute and chronic inflammatory changes occur within weeks or a few months after ileostomy closure. Partial villous atrophy is seen in 60% of patients at 6 weeks, with an initial reduction occurring within 5 days. Changes include a diminution in villous/total mucosal thickness ratio, a fall in the intraepithelial lymphocyte population and a small increase in CD3 positive cells within the lamina propria at 5 days. Haemotoxylin and eosin-based grading, and human leukocyte antigen (HLA)-DR expression remain unchanged. There is little evidence of increased macrophage infiltration over this period. An immune mechanism is possible but is not supported by these observations, and the early morphological changes observed following ileostomy closure suggest the influence of an intraluminal factor likely to involve faecal metabolism.

Comparison of morphological studies following restorative proctocolectomy in patients with ulcerative colitis and FAP show that, whilst the degree of villous atrophy and the intra-epithelial CD4/CD8 ratio are unchanged, intraepithelial lymphocyte counts are reduced and the labelling index estimated by Ki67 expression and lamina propria cytokine mRNA expression are increased in patients with colitis compared with those with polyposis. Bioassay of leukotriene N4 and prostaglandin E_2 within mucosal biopsies taken from the ileal pouch in patients with ulcerative colitis or polyposis, also show differences even in temporarily defunctioned patients, indicating that a systemic disease-related factor may be important.[54]

An increased prevalence of pouchitis in colitic patients affected with primary sclerosing cholangitis (PSC) has been reported.[55] At a follow-up of 6 years from closure of ileostomy, approximately 70% of patients with PSC had pouchitis compared with a prevalence of pouchitis of just over 40% in those not affected by PSC.

Current smokers appear to have significantly fewer episodes of pouchitis than either non-smokers or former smokers.[56]

Further work is required to identify the cellular and molecular events occurring after faecal contact with ileal pouch mucosa following ileostomy reversal. There is evidence that faecal composition plays a role in inducing mucosal inflammation. However, this is not the only factor given the similar levels of mediators observed in defunctioned and functioning colitic ileal pouches. A possible genetic propensity requires further research. The response of pouchitis to metronidazole supports a microbiological factor. The relationship of pouchitis to smoking and PSC indicates biological effects similar to ulcerative colitis as do the histological appearances and the overwhelming relationship of pouchitis to the group of patients having restorative proctocolectomy for ulcerative colitis.

Clinical Presentation

Most patients have a marked increase of frequency and fluidity of the stool. They may also have activity related extraintestinal manifestations, such as arthralgia, skin rashes and episcleritis.[8,57]

There appear to be two distinct forms of the condition. The acute presentation responds rapidly to metronidazole, whilst chronic pouchitis does not do so and is unlikely to respond to conventional anti-inflammatory medication. Some of these cases may be difficult to distinguish from Crohn's disease.

The clinical subdivision into acute, acute relapsing and chronic unremitting is supported by clinicopathological studies, where 60 patients were followed up for a median period of 8.3 years. Of these, 45% never developed pouchitis and had no histological evidence of acute inflammation at any time, 13% had chronic unremitting pouchitis, and the remaining 42% had either acute or acute relapsing pouchitis. These groups were distinguishable on biopsy examination at 3–6 months and hence may provide an early means of identifying patients at risk of developing chronic unremitting pouchitis. It has also been suggested by some groups that chronic unremitting pouchitis may be more common in males. Similar observations have been made by Verres et al.[58]

Histology

Chronic Inflammation and Villous Atrophy. Acute inflammation is seen with neutrophil infiltration of the muscularis mucosa. Chronic lymphocyte infiltrate may also be seen with epithelial mucosal breaks (Fig. 1.6). Additionally, fibromuscular obliteration of the lamina propria and crypt hyperplasia may be seen. However, caution should be exercised in interpreting such atrophy, and crypt hyperplasia may be a normal feature of healthy pelvic ileal pouches. The inflammatory infiltrate may be graded and the more severe grades correlate closely with endoscopic appearance and frequency of defaecation.[59,60] There is also correlation with the degree of villous atrophy which is itself related to the degree of crypt

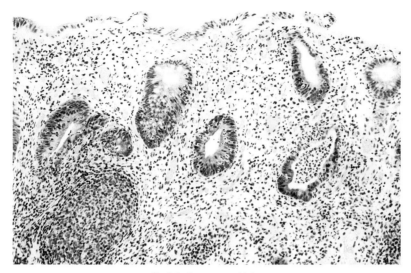

Fig. 1.6. Severe pouchitis.

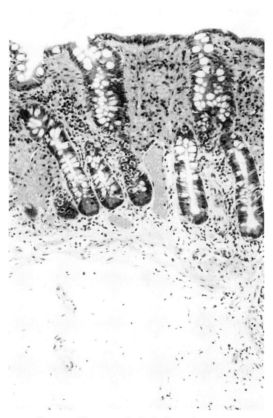

Fig. 1.7. Villous atrophy in ileal pouch mucosa.

hyperplasia, epithelial cell renewal and frequency of defaecation (Fig. 1.7). However, inflammation does not appear to be related to pouch design efficiency or pouch emptying, or age of the patient.

Colonic Metaplasia. Histologically the presence of severe villous atrophy and crypt hyperplasia resembles colonic mucosa. When inflammation is present the picture looks like ulcerative colitis: studies have shown colonic type mucin in ileal pouches irrespective of the original diagnosis.[61] Using Alcian blue staining techniques and the monoclonal PR3A5, which is thought to be specific for colon-type mucin, the presence of sulphated mucin has been demonstrated in ileal pouch mucosa.[62] A similar result has been reported using a S^3H glucosamine-labelling technique.[61] However, these changes are not complete. For example, the pouch mucosa retains certain properties of small intestinal enterocytes with preservation of disaccharidase and the ability to absorb B_{12} xylose and bile acids. It is not known whether colonic metaplasia is a prerequisite for pouchitis.

"Diversion" Changes. In defunctioned pouches prior to closure of the ileostomy histological abnormalities have been reported in a proportion of patients.[63] These include villous atrophy, chronic inflammation with eosinophil predominance, and acute inflammation. The changes are not typical of ischaemia or Crohn's disease and may represent a form of diversion ileitis analogous to that described in the colon and rectum.

Microbiology

Although stool culture is usually performed it is often unhelpful, the exceptions are if either *Clostridium difficile*[64] or *Salmonella* are grown, which may be rare differential diagnoses and respond to specific therapy (metronidazole, ciprofloxacin or vancomycin).

Leukocyte Scintigraphy

[111]Indium-labelled leukocytes administered intravenously and then scanned in a gamma counter produce a characteristic appearance in the pouch. This may be useful for diagnosing patchy disease.[65] Scans have a sensitivity of 70% and a specificity of about 80% and both the scan index and faecal excretion of labelled white blood cells fall rapidly with metronidazole therapy.

Calproctectin

Calproctectin is a stable product of polymorpholeukocyte breakdown. Faecal concentrations and 24-hour output estimation correlate significantly with the severity of inflammation in the ileal mucosa judged histopathologically.[66]

Crohn's Disease

Crohn's disease represents a relatively small percentage of patients with pouch inflammation. Review of the initial colectomy specimen is important in making a diagnosis, but granulomas from the pouch biopsy may be due to a foreign body reaction to particulate matter in the lumen or to mucin. Anal fissures may be non-specific. Granulomas may be present in the pouch of patients with an incontestable diagnosis of ulcerative colitis,[67] hence Crohn's disease should not be diagnosed on this basis alone without a careful review of the histology from the original operative specimen and an assessment of clinical and radiological features.

Treatment

Medical. Attention should be given to symptomatic relief with anti-diarrhoeals and replacement of iron and vitamins.

Metronidazole appears to be effective in about 80% of patients. Its mode of action is largely as an anti-anaerobic agent but it also may inhibit superoxide production and hence toxic oxygen derived free radical induced mucosal damage.[68] Some groups have used the response to metronidazole as a diagnostic test of pouchitis but clearly up to 20% of cases (often chronic) will not respond. The usual dose is 200 mg orally thrice daily. Topical 5-ASA enemas may also be useful in pouchitis but no randomised control trial evidence is available. Chronic pouchitis may respond to oral 5-ASA derivatives. While topical steroids in the form of suppositories or enemas may produce a symptomatic improvement, systemic steroids may be used if patients are ill, febrile or exhibit extraintestinal manifestations. Cyclosporin A retention enemas have been tried with mixed success in refractory pouchitis.[57]

Anecdotal evidence is available of the efficacy of kaopectate, a resin that binds endotoxin, improving pouchitis.[69]

There have been some anecdotal reports of the topical administration of short-chain fatty acids and the amino acid glutamine, which are known to be the predominant luminal nutrients for colonocytes and enterocytes respectively.[70,71] The apparent early benefit of these substances in the treatment of chronic pouchitis warrants further study.

Surgical. Surgery may be necessary although in practice this is uncommon.[72] Simple defunctioning will relieve frequency of defaecation but does not influence the intensity of the inflammation. A temporary ileostomy is unlikely to be reversed at a later date. A few patients require pouch excision although in several series this has been reported as being around 1% of patients with pouchitis.[52]

Neoplastic Transformation

When dysplasia is present, a full rectal excision should be carried out. A mucosectomy of dysplastic rectal mucosa is not indicated since there may be microinvasion. The cases of carcinoma in the denuded rectal stump reported by Stern et al.[73] and von Herbay et al.[74] are probably examples of this.

Low-grade dysplasia in the ileal pouch in a small group of patients with previous ulcerative colitis has been reported by Verres et al.[78] This was found in those with unremitting chronic and acute inflammation of the ileal mucosa from the outset following ileostomy closure. Medium term follow up (8±5 years) in 60 patients followed by regular biopsies during the period, did not show any case of dysplasia.[52] However, it is important to follow patients indefinitely to determine the long-term outcome concerning transformation.

So far, to the authors' knowledge, there has been no case of invasive malignancy in an ileoanal pouch in a colitic patient, but this has now occurred in a Kock reservoir.[76]

In FAP, adenoma formation in the pouch is common,[77,78] occurring in 13% and 42% respectively over a median follow-up period of 4 and 5 years. Very rarely, invasive carcinoma can arise from the small intestine of FAP patients,[79,80] and there has been one report of this occurring in an ileal pouch 3 years after restorative proctocolectomy.[81] The long-term incidence of invasive neoplasia in the pouch in FAP is not known, but continued surveillance in this disease is clearly essential.

References

1. Dozois RR, Goldberg SM, Rothenberger DA et al. (1986) Restorative proctocolectomy with ileal reservoir. Int J Colorectal Dis 1:2–19.
2. Cohen Z, McLeod RS, Stephen W, Stern HS, Reznick R (1985) The pelvic pouch and ileoanal anastomosis procedure: surgical procedure and initial results. Am J Surg 150:601–607.
3. Nicholls RJ (1987) Restorative proctocolectomy with various types of reservoir. World J Surg 11:751–762.
4. Pemberton JH, Kelly KA, Beart RW, Dozois RR, Wolff BG, Ilstrup DM (1987) Ileal pouch-anal anastomosis for chronic ulcerative colitis. Long-term results. Ann Surg 206:504–513.
5. Fazio VW, Ziv Y, Church JM et al. (1995) Ileal pouch-anal anastomoses complications and function in 1005 patients. Ann Surg 222(2):120–127.
6. Bauer JJ, Gorfine SR, Gelernt IM, Harris MT, Kreel I (1997) Restorative proctocolectomy in patients older than fifty years. Dis Colon Rectum 40:562–565.
7. Dayton MT, Larsen KR (1996) Should older patients undergo ileal pouch-anal anastomosis? Am J Surg 172:444–447; discussion 447–448.
8. Setti-Carraro P, Ritchie JK, Wilkinson KH, Nicholls RJ, Hawley PR (1994) The first 10 years' experience of restorative proctocolectomy for ulcerative colitis. Gut 35:1070–1075.
9. Panis Y, Poupard B, Nemeth J, Lavergne A, Hautefeuille P, Valleur P (1996) Ileal pouch/anal anastomosis for Crohn's disease. Lancet 347:854–857.
10. Price AB (1978) Overlap in the spectrum of non-specific inflammatory bowel disease – "colitis indeterminate". J Clin Pathol 31:567–577.
11. Wells AD, McMillan I, Price AB, Ritchie JK, Nicholls RJ (1991) Natural history of indeterminate colitis. Br J Surg 78:179–181.
12. Pezim ME, Pemberton JH, Beart RWJ et al. (1989) Outcome of "indeterminant" colitis following ileal pouch-anal anastomosis. Dis Colon Rectum 32:653–658.
13. Koltun W, Schoetz DJ, Roberts PL, Murray JJ, Coller JA, Veidenheimer MC (1990) Indeterminate colitis predisposes to perineal complications after ileal pouch-anal anastomosis. Dis Colon Rectum 33:4.
14. Korsgen S, Keighley MR (1997) Causes of failure and life expectancy of the ileoanal pouch. Int J Colorectal Dis 12:4–8.
15. Lewis WG, Sagar PM, Holdsworth PJ et al. (1993) Restorative proctocolectomy with end to end pouch-anal anastomosis in patients over the age of fifty. Gut 34:948–952.
16. Seow-Choen F, Ho YH, Goh HS (1994) The ileo-anal reservoir: results from an evolving use of stapling devices. J R Coll Surg Edinb 39:13–16.
17. Hallgren TA, Fasth SB, Oresland TO, Hulten LA (1995) Ileal pouch anal function after endoanal mucosectomy and handsewn ileoanal anastomosis compared with stapled anastomosis without mucosectomy [see comments]. Eur J Surg 161:915–921.
18. Nicholls RJ, Pezim ME (1985) Restorative proctocolectomy with ileal reservoir for UC and FAP: a comparison of 3 reservoir designs. Br J Surg 72:470–474.

19. Lazorthes F, Fages P, Chiotasso P, Lenozy J, Bloom E (1986) Resection of the rectum with construction of a colonic reservoir and colo-anal anastomosis for carcinoma of the rectum. Br J Surg 73:136–138.
20. Kock NG, Hulten L, Myrvold HE (1989) Ileoanal anastomosis with interposition of the ileal "Kock pouch". Dis Colon Rectum 32:1050–1054.
21. Pescatori M, Manhire A, Bartram CI (1983) Evacuation pouchography in the evaluation of ileoanal reservoir function. Dis Colon Rectum 26:365–368.
22. Lavery IC, Sirimarco MT, Ziv Y, Fazio VW (1995) Anal canal inflammation after ileal pouch-anal anastomosis. The need for treatment. Dis Colon Rectum 38:803–806.
23. Lee ECG, Dowling BL (1972) Perimuscular excision of the rectum for Crohn's disease and ulcerative colitis. Br J Surg 59:29–43.
24. Berry AR, de Campos R, Lee EC (1986) Perineal and pelvic morbidity following perimuscular excision of the rectum for inflammatory bowel disease. Br J Surg 73:675–677.
25. Keenan RA (1994) Ileostomy "twist" – an avoidable complication [letter; comment]. Dis Colon Rectum 37:1176–1177.
26. Becker JM, Dayton MT, Fazio VW et al. (1996) Prevention of postoperative abdominal adhesions by a sodium hyaluronate-based bioresorbable membrane: a prospective, randomized, double-blind multicenter study [see comments]. J Am Coll Surg 183:297–306.
27. Beck DE(1997) The role of Seprafilm bioresorbable membrane in adhesion prevention. Eur J Surg [Suppl] 577:49–55.
28. Madden MV, Neale KF, Nicholls RJ et al. (1991) Comparison of morbidity and function after colectomy with ileorectal anastomosis or restorative proctocolectomy for familial adenomatous polyposis. Br J Surg 78:789–792.
29. Thow GB (1985) Single-stage colectomy and mucosal proctectomy with stapled antiperistaltic ileoanal reservoir. In: Dozois RR (ed) Alternatives to conventional ileostomy. Year Book Medical, Chicago, pp 420–432.
30. Everett WG (1989) Experience of restorative proctocolectomy with ileal reservoir. Br J Surg 76:77–81.
31. Grobler SP, Hosie KB, Keighley MRB (1992)Randomized trial of loop ileostomy in restorative proctocolectomy. Br J Surg 79:903–906.
32. Senapati A, Nicholls RJ, Ritchie JK, Tibbs CJ, Hawley PR (1993)Temporary loop ileostomy for restorative proctocolectomy. Br J Surg 80:628–630.
33. Winslet MC, Barsoum G, Pringle W, Fox K, Keighley MR (1991) Loop ileostomy after ileal pouch-anal anastomosis – is it necessary? Dis Colon Rectum 34:267–270.
34. Ozuner G, Hull T, Lee P, Fazio VW (1997) What happens to a pelvic pouch when a fistula develops? Dis Colon Rectum 40:543–547.
35. Wong WD, Rothenberger DA, Goldberg SM (1985) Ileoanal pouch procedures. Curr Probl Surg 22:1–78.
36. Wexner SD, Rothenberger DA, Jensen L et al. (1989) Ileal pouch-vaginal fistulas: incidence, aetiology and management. Dis Colon Rectum 32:460–465.
37. Oresland T, Fasth S, Nordgren S, Hulten L (1989) The clinical and functional outcome after restorative proctocolectomy. A prospective study in 100 patients. Int J Colorectal Dis 4:50–56.
38. Keighley MRB, Asperer J, Hosie K, Grobler S (1991) Fistula complicating restorative proctocolectomy. Gut 32:A557.
39. Groom JS, Nicholls RJ, Hawley PR, Phillips RK (1993) Pouch-vaginal fistula. Br J Surg 80:936–940.
40. Fleshman JW, McLeod RS, Cohen Z, Stern H (1988) Improved results following use of an advancement technique in the treatment of ileoanal anastomotic complications. Int J Colorectal Dis 3:161–165.
41. O'Kelly TJ, Merrett M, Mortensen NJ, Dehn TC, Kettlewell M (1994) Pouch-vaginal fistula after restorative proctocolectomy: aetiology and management. Br Journal Surg 81:1374–1375.
42. Lee PY, Fazio VW, Church JM, Hull TL, Eu KW, Lavery IC (1997) Vaginal fistula following restorative proctocolectomy. Dis Colon Rectum 40:752–759.
43. Hughes LE, Donaldson DR, Williams JG, Taylor BA, Young HL (1988) Local depot methylprednisolone injection for painful anal Crohn's disease. Gastroenterology 94:709–711.
44. Senapati A, Tibbs CJ, Ritchie JK, Nicholls RJ, Hawley PR (1996) Stenosis of the pouch anal anastomosis following restorative proctocolectomy. Int J Colorectal Dis 11:57–59.
45. Galandiuk S, Scott NA, Dozois RR et al. (1990) Ileal pouch-anal anastomosis. Reoperation for pouch-related complications. Ann Surg 212:446–452.
46. Herbst F, Sielezneff I, Nicholls RJ (1996) Salvage surgery for ileal pouch outlet obstruction. Br J Surg 83:368–371.

47. Korsgen S, Nikiteas N, Ogunbiyi OA, Keighley MR (1996) Results from pouch salvage. Br J Surg 83:372–374.
48. Nicholls RJ, Gilbert JM (1990) Surgical correction of the efferent ileal limb for disordered defae-cation following restorative proctocolectomy with the S ileal reservoir. Br J Surg 77:152–154.
49. Hull TL, Fazio VW, Schroeder T (1995) Paradoxical puborectalis contraction in patients after pelvic pouch construction. Dis Colon Rectum 38:1144–1146.
50. Ravitch MM, Sabiston DC (1947) Anal ileostomy with preservation of the sphincter. Surg Gynecol Obstet 84:1095–1099.
51. Heppel J, Kelly KA, Phillips SP, Beart RW, Telander RL, Perrault J (1947) Physiologic aspects of continence after colectomy, mucosal proctocolectomy and endorectal ileo-anal anastomosis. Ann Surg 195:435–443.
52. Setti Carraro P, Talbot IC, Nicholls RJ (1994) Longterm appraisal of the histological appearances of the ileal reservoir mucosa after restorative proctocolectomy for ulcerative colitis. Gut 35:1721–1727.
53. Apel R, Cohen Z, Andrews CW, McLeod RS, Steinhart H, Odze RD (1994) Prospective evaluation of early morphological changes in pelvic pouches. Gastroenterology 107:435–443.
54. Gertner DJ, Rampton DS, Madden MV, Talbot IC, Nicholls RJ, Lennard-Jones JE (1994) Increased leukotriene B$_4$ release from ileal pouch mucosa in ulcerative colitis compared with familial ade-nomatous polyposis. Gut 35:1429–1432.
55. Penna C, Dozois R, Tremaine W et al. (1996) Pouchitis after ileal pouch-anal anastomosis for ulcerative colitis occurs with increased frequency in patients with associated primary sclerosing cholangitis. Gut 38:234–239.
56. Merrett MN, Mortensen N, Kettlewell M, Jewell DP (1996) Smoking may prevent pouchitis in patients with restorative proctocolectomy for ulcerative colitis. Gut 38:362–364.
57. Lohmuller JL, Pemberton JH, Dozois RR, Ilstrup D, van Heerden J (1990) Pouchitis and extrain-testinal manifestation of inflammatory bowel disease after ileal pouch-anal anastomosis. Ann Surg 211:622–629.
58. Verres B, Reinholt FP, Lindquist K, Liljeqvist L (1992) Mucosal adaptation in the ileal reservoir after restorative proctocolectomy. A long term follow up study. Ann Chir 46:10–18.
59. Moskowitz RL, Shepherd NA, Nicholls RJ (1986) Inflammation in the reservoir after restorative proctocolectomy with ileal reservoir. Int J Colorectal Dis 1:167–174.
60. Kmiot WA, Youngs D, Tudor R, Thompson H, Keighley MR (1993) Mucosal morphology, cell pro-liferation and faecal bacteriology in acute pouchitis. Br J Surg 80:1445–1449.
61. Corfield AP, Warren BF, Bartolo DCC (1990) Colonic metaplasia following restorative procto-colectomy monitored using a new metabolic labelling technique for mucin. J Pathol 160:170A.
62. de Silva HJ, Gatter KC, Millard PR, Kettlewell M, Mortensen N, Jewell DP (1990) Crypt cell prolif-eration and HLA DR expression in pelvic ileal pouches. J Clin Pathol 43:824–828.
63. Meuwissen SCM, Hoitsma H, Boot H, Seldenrijk CA (1989) Pouchitis (pouch ileitis). Neth J Med 35:554–556.
64. Madden MV, McIntyre AS, Nicholls RJ (1994) Double-blind crossover trial of metronidazole versus placebo in chronic unremitting pouchitis. Dig Dis Sci 39:1193–1196.
65. Kmiot WA, Hesslewood SR, Smith N, Thompson H, Harding LK, Keighley MR (1993) Evaluation of the inflammatory infiltrate in pouchitis with ^{111}In-labeled granulocytes. Gastroenterology 104:981–988.
66. Winter TA, Dalton HR, Merrett MN, Campbell A, Jewell DP (1993) Cyclosporin A retention enemas in refractory distal ulcerative colitis and 'pouchitis'. Scand J Gastroenterol 28:701–704.
67. Shepherd NA, Jass JR, Duval I, Moskowitz RL, Nicholls RJ, Morson BC (1987) Restorative procto-colectomy with ileal reservoir: pathological and histochemical study of mucosal biopsy speci-mens. J Clin Pathol 40:601–607.
68. Levin KE, Pemberton JH, Phillips SF, Zinsmeister AR, Pezim ME (1992) Role of oxygen free radi-cals in the aetiology of pouchitis. Dis Colon Rectum 35:452–456.
69. Keighley MR. The management of pouchitis. Aliment Pharmacol Ther 10:449–457.
70. den Hoed PT, van Goch JJ, Veen HF, Ouwendijk RJ (1996) Severe pouchitis successfully treated with short-chain fatty acids. Can J Surg 39:168–169 (letter).
71. Wischmeyer P, Pemberton JH, Phillips SF (1993) Chronic pouchitis after ileal pouch-anal anasto-mosis: responses to butyrate and glutamine suppositories in a pilot study. Mayo Clin Proc 68:978–981.
72. Marcello PW, Roberts PL, Schoetz DJ Jr, Coller JA, Murray JJ, Veidenheimer MC (1993) Long-term results of the ileoanal pouch procedure. Arch of Surg 128:500–503; discussion 503–504.
73. Stern H, Walfish S, Mullen B, McLeod R, Cohen Z (1990) Cancer in an ileoanal reservoir: a new late complication? Gut 31:473–475.

74. von Herbay A, Stern J, Herfarth C (1996) Pouch-anal cancer after restorative proctocolectomy for familial adenomatous polyposis. Am J Surg Pathol 20:995–999.
75. Verres B, Reinholt FP, Lindquist K, Lofberg R, Liljeqvist L (1995) Long-term histomorphological surveillance of the pelvic ileal pouch: dysplasia develops in a subgroup of patients. Gastroenterology 109:1090–1097.
76. Cox CL, Butts DR, Roberts MP, Wessels RA, Bailey HR (1997) Development of invasive adeno-carcinoma in a long-standing Kock continent ileostomy: report of a case. Dis Colon Rectum 40:500–503.
77. Nugent KP, Spigelman AD, Nicholls RJ, Talbot IC, Neale K, Phillips RKS (1993) Pouch adenomas in patients with familial adenomatous polyposis. Br J Surg 80:1620.
78. Wu JS, McGannon EA, Church JM (1998) Incidence of neoplastic polyps in the ileal pouch of patients with familial adenomatous polyposis after restorative proctocolectomy. Dis Colon Rectum 41:552–557.
79. Primrose JN, Quirke P, Johnston D (1988) Carcinoma of the ileostomy in a patient with familial adenomatous polyposis. Br J Surg 75:384.
80. Gilson TP, Sollenberger LL (1992) Adenocarcinoma of an ileostomy in a patient with familial adenomatous polyposis. Dis Colon Rectum 35:261–265.
81. Bassuini MM, Billings PJ (1996) Carcinoma in an ileoanal pouch after restorative proctocolectomy for familial adenomatous polyposis. Br J Surg 83:506.

2 Laparoscopic Colorectal Surgery

M.R. Salum and S.D. Wexner

Introduction

The advent and reportedly positive results of laparoscopic cholecystectomy[1-3] along with advances in instrumentation has prompted surgeons to apply laparoscopic techniques to the treatment of other gastrointestinal diseases including disorders of the colon, rectum and anus.

The first laparoscopic appendectomy was performed by DeKok in 1977.[4] This laparoscopic–assisted procedure included a minilaparotomy to remove the uninflamed appendix. Semm[5] achieved the first complete laparoscopic appendectomy in 1983. Laparoscopy subsequently became practical and popular among both general and gynaecological surgeons for the evaluation and treatment of right lower quadrant pain in women.[6,7]

Initially the application of the laparoscopic technique for colorectal surgery was limited due to the lack of appropriate instrumentation. Therefore the first published laparoscopic colon resection was in fact a laparoscopic-assisted procedure. Subsequently the introduction of laparoscopic intestinal staplers made it possible for virtually all types of colorectal procedures to be completely accomplished through the laparoscope.

Justification for Laparoscopic Colorectal Surgery

Some early retrospective reports failed to find significant advantages after colectomies performed by laparoscopic technique when compared with standard laparotomy.[8-11] The only consistent initially accepted benefit of laparoscopy in colorectal surgery has been improved cosmesis.[9,12,13] Ultimately, however, even this benefit has come into question by those investigators who have shown that cosmesis is a very subjective issue and found no statistically significant differences relative to cosmesis between laparoscopy and laparotomy.[14]

Some of the parameters used to assess the efficacy of these procedures include the length of hospitalisation and the patient's ability to return to a normal lifestyle. Indeed, length of stay has reportedly decreased after laparoscopic colorectal surgery compared with conventional colorectal surgery.[15-19]

Decreasing the length of postoperative ileus can contribute to shorter hospital stay. It has been hypothesised that laparoscopic colorectal surgery, because of less trauma and manipulation of the bowel, results in earlier recovery of bowel

function. One animal study[20] clearly shows an earlier return of bowel myoelectri-
cal activity and normal bowel movement after laparoscopy compared with conventional right colectomy. Whether this benefit is actual or simply perceived in
humans is unknown. It would be difficult to prove any advantage relative to return
of gut function and laparoscopy as almost all patients who undergo laparoscopic
colectomy can tolerate oral intake within 24 hours of surgery.

Thus early return of bowel function may not be a unique attribute of laparoscopic surgery. Binderow et al.[21] and Reissman et al.[22] have shown in two separate
prospective randomised trials of over 200 patients that the ability to tolerate oral
intake in the early postoperative period is not exclusive to laparoscopy.
Approximately 89% of patients can tolerate a diet within one day of laparotomy
and colectomy.

In evaluating decreased pain as a potential benefit to the laparoscopic
approach, Ramos et al. [23] showed that patients who underwent laparotomy used
patient-controlled analgesia for 6.2 days postoperatively versus 2.9 days if the procedure was done laparoscopically. Many other more recent studies have confirmed
these findings.

In addition to conferring some distinct advantages, the total charges involved
in laparoscopy and laparotomy have not been found to differ significantly. Both
Reiver et al.[24] and Falk et al.[25] demonstrated that although the operating room
charges (largely due to disposable instruments) was greater for laparoscopy, the
mean hospital stay was significantly shorter, therefore the overall charges were
similar in both groups. Senagore et al.[26] reported that their overall charges were
actually lower for patients who underwent laparoscopy. They attributed the
savings not only to reduction of hospital stay, but also to the use of fewer phar-
maceutical agents, intravenous infusions and intramuscular injections as compared with laparotomy.

Multiple attempts have been made to assess at the true charges associated with
laparoscopic surgery. Limitations have resulted from inadequate cost assessment
techniques and lack of standardisation of the parameters used to define cost.
Despite these limitations, almost all studies have determined that the operative
costs are higher for laparoscopic cases. This finding is due to longer operating
room time and the use of additional disposable and non-disposable equipment
compared with laparotomy. The total cost is especially higher for laparoscopic
cases that must be converted to laparotomy. Total cost saving is possible if the
patient's hospital stay is shortened or the patient returns to productive activity in
a shorter time period. However, economic pressures and newer management
principles including day of surgery admission, early postoperative feeding and
home health care have lowered the length of hospitalisation associated with
laparotomy. Increased use of reusable instruments and shorter operating times
may further reduce the total cost of laparoscopy.

It is apparent that there is a steep learning curve associated with laparoscopic
colorectal surgery.[27] It requires more skill and presents more challenging issues
than does most other laparoscopic surgery. There exist several differences
between laparoscopic colorectal surgery and most other laparoscopic procedures.
First, while all other laparoscopic procedures involve one main anatomical region,
the laparoscopic technique for colon resection requires dissection and mobilisation in more than one region. To obtain the best operating field the surgeon often
has to change the position of the camera, instruments, and even of the personnel
during the procedure. To aid dissection, the mobilised bowel needs to be

retracted; however, this manoeuvre is not easily accomplished within the confined space of the abdominal cavity, often resulting in long, tedious surgery.

Other features unique to colorectal surgery are ligation of vessels and removal of a large specimen. Mesenteric vessels are numerous, large, often calcified and course in a thick layer of opaque fat. Laparoscopically isolating these pedicles and subsequently ligating and dividing them can be much more difficult than during laparotomy. Most recently, the use of the harmonic scalpel (Ethicon Endosurgery Inc., Cincinnati, Ohio) has conferred a definite advantage in mesenteric dissection and vascular control by allowing adequate haemostasis without the decreased visibility associated with the smoke created by extensive electrocoagulation. To effect removal of specimens, incisions of up to 25 cm have been made, thereby limiting the cosmetic benefit.[28] Specimen bags have been made available to decrease contamination by bacteria or tumour when the specimen is negotiated through a small wound.

An integral part of most colonic resections is fashioning an anastomosis. To achieve a well-vascularised, tension-free, circumferentially intact anastomosis the surgeon needs infinite patience and experience. Nevertheless, Phillips et al.[18], in their report of 51 laparoscopic low anterior resections, noted that the circular stapled anastomosis was incomplete in 18% of cases. This extraordinarily high rate of incomplete anastomosis compares poorly with the 2–8% rate during laparotomy.[29] The development of the endoscopic linear cutting device (Ethicon Endosurgery Inc.) may have reduced the need for this step but at a greater cost.

General Considerations

Preoperative preparation is similar to that used for laparotomy.[30] Patients are given a mechanical bowel preparation with 90 cc of sodium phosphate-based oral solutions (Fleet's phosphosoda; C.B. Fleet, Lynchburg, Va.), which has been demonstrated in a prospective fashion to be more tolerable for patients than the "standard" 4 litre sodium phosphate preparation.[31] Both parenteral and oral antibiotics are given prior to the operation; all patients are asked for their consent for a laparotomy and for intraoperative colonoscopy. Antithrombotic measures such as heparin or enoxoparin sodium and sequential compression stockings are utilised. After the induction of general endotracheal anaesthesia, a nasogastric tube and an indwelling bladder catheter are placed to minimise the risk of trocar injury to the stomach and bladder, respectively. The patient is placed in the supine modified lithotomy position in Allen stirrups (Allen Medical, Bedford Heights, Ohio). Flexion at the hips and knees should be limited to no greater than 15% to allow for ease of instrument movement. This position allows more flexibility for the surgeon, assistant, camera operator, and permits colonoscopy.

The abdomen is prepared and draped in the standard fashion to provide wide exposure in case a laparotomy is necessary. The patient is then placed in a steep Trendelenburg position and a 1-cm transverse incision is made either above or below the umbilicus. Pneumoperitoneum is usually established by using a Veress needle. In patients in whom previous surgery has been performed, an "open" Hasson technique may be used.[32] The Veress needle is introduced and correct placement is verified in four ways. First, the surgeon should have the manual tactile sense that the needle has entered the peritoneal cavity. Second, an audible noise should be appreciated as the needle enters the abdominal cavity. Third, a few millilitres of sterile water are placed on top of the vertically held needle conus. By lifting the anterior abdominal wall, the surgeon creates negative intra-abdominal pressure and the liquid is drawn into the abdominal cavity. Finally, high-flow insufflation should result in a gradual rise in the intra-abdominal pressure. A rapid rise or appearance of subcutaneous crepitus indicates preperitoneal needle placement. After the pneumoperitoneum is established with carbon dioxide to a pressure of 15 mmHg the Veress needle is removed and a 10/12-mm trocar is placed through this umbilical port site. The zero degree camera is then introduced through the port and all subsequent work is undertaken under direct endoscopic visualisation.

Another consideration in patients after previous pelvic surgery is the insertion of ureteric catheters. Either ordinary or illuminated stents may expedite the identification of the ureters during a laparoscopic procedure in the presence of multiple adhesions and distorted anatomy. Indications for stents include inflammatory conditions, or prior pelvic surgery, sepsis or radiation.

All cannulas are 10–12 mm in diameter to enable flexibility of instruments and camera relocation as dictated by the anatomical findings. The number of ports used may vary between three and five, according to the procedure performed. Three ports are commonly used for stoma creation and three, four and rarely even five may be required for resection. As the procedure progresses, some cannulas are replaced with a larger size (18 or 33 mm) using a Seldinger technique with a 10-mm exchange rod (Ethicon Endosurgery Inc.) This manoeuvre enables the use of both linear and circular stapler devices and facilitates specimen retrieval. Frequent relocation of personnel and instruments may be required during the procedure to facilitate dissection in different abdominal quadrants. Frequent alterations in the patient's position, such as Trendelenburg, reverse Trendelenburg and tilt to the sides, may improve exposure of the surgical field.

The more commonly used instruments for laparoscopy include Babcock clamps, Denis (non-crushing) bowel clamps, 10 mm diameter scissors, Kelly clamps, right-angled and modified Allis clamps, short (35 mm) and long (60 mm) linear stapler devices, circular 29–33 mm stapler devices, 10–12, 18 and 33 mm cannulas, bowel retractors, endoloops, endoclips and a hernia stapler. The last-mentioned instrument can be employed for either closure of the mesenteric defect or marking of the planned resection margins.[33] More recently almost all of the dissection and mobilisation has been undertaken with the harmonic scalpel (Ethicon Endosurgery Inc.).

As with laparotomy, most procedures usually begin with mobilisation of the bowel through gentle traction and countertraction. Positioning of the patient facilitates retraction by using gravity to move the bowel away from the field of vision.[34] A significant limitation with laparoscopy is the surgeon's loss of tactile sensation. Exact identification of lesions by palpation is impossible and the mere assumption of the position based on preoperative colonoscopy has led to the inadvertent removal of wrong segments of bowel. At initial colonoscopy, the endoscopist can mark the lesion with India ink, indigo carmine, indocyanine green or methylene blue to allow visualisation during laparoscopy. A preoperative air–contrast barium enema can also facilitate exact anatomic definition. If the site of the lesion is in doubt, an intraoperative colonoscopy can identify the location of the lesion. A non–crushing laparoscopic clamp (Endopath clamp; Ethicon Endosurgery Inc.) is used to prevent air insufflation into the small bowel during colonoscopy. The site of the lesion may be marked with a clip, suture or electrocautery and the colonoscope is then withdrawn along with any residual air. These manoeuvres will help to avoid the removal of the wrong segment of bowel.[8,35-37]

Once the colon is mobilised, attention is directed to the ligation of vessels, which can be done either extra or intracorporeally. With extracorporeal ligation, an incision is made, the bowel is then eviscerated through this usually 3- to 5-cm-long incision along with its previously mobilised mesentery. The vessels are then ligated in the standard fashion.

If intracorporeal ligation is preferred or mandated because of a shortened mesentery, several methods are available. A vascular stapling device, similar to that used for the bowel, with modified clip sizes, can be applied to ligate the vessels. This procedure, however, adds to the procedure's cost. Alternatively, a less expensive method involves meticulous dissection of the vascular pedicles with independent clipping or even ligation of vessels with an endoscopic loop. This dissection, however, is significantly more difficult, potentially more dangerous, and definitely more time-consuming. The harmonic scalpel (Ethicon Endosurgery Inc.) facilitates haemostatic, relatively expedient, mesenteric division. Technically, the resection margins, mesenteric excision and height of vascular ligation can equal those of laparotomy.[38] Again, the surgeon has the option of performing the anastomosis either extra- or intracorporeally. If extracorporeal resection and anastomosis is performed, conventional methods are applied. This laparoscopic-assisted technique is most suitable for right hemicolectomy. The caecum and the ascending colon are mobilised along the white line of Toldt to the midline. A variable amount of the hepatic flexure and proximal transverse colon are mobilised as well. A small incision is made by extending the site of the umbilical port, which may then be used to lift the abdominal wall, insulating the bowel below from the cautery. The right colon is gently removed and resection, vascular ligation, anastomosis and mesenteric defect closure are effected. Alternatively, right-sided anastomosis can be completely intracorporeally performed with an endoscopic linear cutting and anastomotic device. This totally laparoscopic procedure can be quite time-consuming, and expensive, requires a great deal of technical expertise and a perfectly prepared bowel. In addition, at least in the setting of right hemicolectomy, the totally laparoscopic technique confers few advantages when compared with the laparoscopic-assisted procedure.[39]

Conversely, left-sided lesions are well suited to an intracorporeal anastomosis, facilitated by a circular stapler.[40] The port site can be incised to the fascia through which the specimen can be removed and the anvil of the circular stapler is placed in the proximal bowel and secured with a pursestring suture. Alternatively, the abdomen can be opened through a Pfannenstiel incision, incorporating the two lowest port sites, through which the procedure is easily completed.

Finally, the same criteria, which apply to laparotomy, should be adhered to for the postoperative phase of laparoscopic colorectal surgery. In our experience, in elective procedures performed by laparotomy or laparoscopy, the nasogastric or orogastric tube may be removed immediately after surgery and a clear liquid diet may be commenced. Almost 90% of patients tolerate a regular diet within 48 hours.[21,22]

Specific Procedures

Laparoscopic Creation of Stoma

Faecal diversion is a relatively common requirement in a colorectal practice and laparoscopic creation of intestinal stomas is both feasible and effective for this purpose.[41] Indications for diversion of stool include faecal incontinence, sphincter injury, fistulae including rectovaginal, colovesical or rectourethral, perineal sepsis due to Crohn's disease or necrotising fasciitis, and radiation proctitis.[42–47]

The operative technique is simple and requires careful preoperative selection of a stoma site by a qualified enterostomal therapist or nurse. This location will also serve as a port site. The initial midline port is placed using either the Veress or Hasson technique. The only caveat for stoma creation is that the camera port should be placed midway between the umbilicus and the xiphoid to prevent interference of the instruments with each other.

After pneumoperitoneum is established the laparoscope is inserted under direct vision; a second 10-mm cannula is placed lateral to the rectus sheath through the stoma site. The surgeon then uses a laparoscopic Babcock-type clamp passed through the stoma site to identify the appropriate loop of bowel and lift it to the stoma site.

For sigmoid colostomy formation, the distal sigmoid, usually draped into the pelvis, is delivered to the anterior abdominal wall. When creating a loop ileostomy, the terminal ileum may not be immediately apparent. However, by grasping and elevating the caecum it comes into view and can be proximally traced from the caecum until an appropriate loop is found that easily reaches the anterior wall. This position is usually 15 to 20 cm proximal to the ileocaecal valve. Placing the patient in steep Trendelenburg position with the left side down can also help in locating the terminal ileum by shifting the overlying small bowel loops into the left upper abdomen. The bowel is gently grasped with the Babcock clamp and brought up to the stoma site cannula. To avoid inadvertent twisting of the bowel, one of several manoeuvres can be utilised to insure appropriate orientation. One technique involves passing a small-bore spinal needle through the abdominal wall medial to the stoma to tattoo the afferent and efferent limbs with methylene blue (one dot proximal and two dots distal) for easy identification. Another effective means of orientation is to perform endoscopy. Alternatively, an instrument can be passed along both the afferent and efferent limbs of the stoma and visualised within by the camera. Finally, a third port can be introduced through which clips can be applied to the mesentery or appendices epiploicae. A combination of these methods may best assure proper orientation. Regardless of which mode is selected, the stoma must be delivered for maturation with appropriate anatomic orientation.

To create the stoma the skin around that port site is excised to allow a 2–3 cm diameter opening. The rectus sheath opening is lengthened by incising along the insulated shaft of the Babcock clamp. The bowel is then withdrawn onto the abdominal wall. With the bowel loop occluding the stoma site, the abdomen is reinsufflated, and the bowel examined once more with the laparoscope to confirm proper orientation. The ostomy is then matured using standard techniques as either an end or a loop stoma.

Appendectomy

Laparoscopic appendectomy is usually performed as an emergency procedure for acute appendicitis or right lower quadrant peritonitis.[48] One of the major advantages of laparoscopic appendectomy over the traditional McBurney incision is the opportunity to perform an exploratory laparoscopy with thorough inspection of the pelvis and the entire abdomen to exclude concomitant or even alternative pathology. This approach has become particularly useful in the diagnosis of right lower quadrant pain in the young female. Salpingitis and tubo-ovarian abscesses are easily diagnosed by laparoscopy and any type of laparotomy and unnecessary appendectomy can be avoided. The patient is prepared in the standard fashion; after pneumoperitoneum is established, the camera is introduced through the periumbilical port and all subsequent work is undertaken under direct vision. After a brief yet thorough exploration of the entire abdominal cavity and pelvis, the diagnosis of acute appendicitis can be confirmed or refuted. If an inflamed appendix is identified, additional trocars can be placed. The second 10/12-mm trocar should be placed in a suprapubic position, below the hairline just cephaled to the symphysis pubis. A third 5-mm trocar should be placed in the right upper quadrant lateral to the rectus muscle. If an additional port is necessary for retraction, it should be 5 mm in size and placed in the right lower quadrant. If the patient has a mobile caecum, an additional port can also be placed in the midline between the first two trocars.

Dissection is initiated by elevating the caecum and identifying the appendix. The distal end of the appendix is retracted laterally and a "window" is made between the vessels in the mesoappendix. Either clips, ligatures, staples or electrocoagulation can be used for securing these vessels. The appendiceal artery should be either proximally secured with two clips or divided with an endoscopic linear cutting stapler.

The stump of the appendix can be managed in a number of ways. Pre-tied vascular sutures can be placed proximally and distally or large haemoclips can be utilised. Usually two clips are placed at the base and the third approximately 2 cm distally to prevent spillage of intraluminal contents; the appendix is then divided with scissors. A more popular and expeditious although expensive method is an endoscopic linear cutting stapler instrument, which may transect both the vessels and the appendix together.

Removal of the appendix can be performed through one of the 10/12-mm trocars or through a plastic bag to lessen the chance of wound contamination and appendiceal rupture.

The trocars should be removed under direct vision to ensure that there is no bleeding or haematoma formation from the port sites. The final umbilical trocar is removed and all incisions are closed. Postoperatively, the nasogastric tube and Foley catheter are removed; the patient should begin to ambulate on the evening of surgery. Antibiotic and pain management is the same as after conventional appendectomy. The diet can be advanced as tolerated, with hospital discharge anticipated generally within 2 to 3 days after surgery.[49]

Sigmoid Colectomy

For sigmoid colectomy three 10/12-mm ports are used: umbilical, right paraumbilical and right lower quadrant. An optional left paraumbilical port may be

needed, especially in obese individuals. Mobilisation of the sigmoid colon can be
facilitated with the patient placed in the steep Trendelenburg position with tilt to
the right. After mobilisation of the colon and identification of the left ureter, the
mesenteric vessels are divided intracorporeally. This division can be performed
with endoclips, vascular stapling devices or the harmonic scalpel (Ethicon
Endosurgery Inc.). After either direct or colonoscopic identification of the lesion,
the distal and proximal margins can be marked with hernia staples. For a tension-
free anastomosis the splenic flexure may need mobilisation; this process is greatly
facilitated by the harmonic scalpel.

For introduction of a 60-mm linear stapler device, the right lower quadrant
10/12-mm port is exchanged for an 18-mm port. The segment of colon previously
marked as the distal margin is then transected. A trial reach of the intended proximal margin is undertaken and that segment is marked with clips. The left
paraumbilical port, if one was used, is replaced with a 33-mm port through which
the proximal colon is gently delivered and the diseased segment is extracorporeally resected. If no left-sided (fourth) port was used then the 33-mm port is introduced de novo. A pursestring suture with a 29- or 33-mm anvil is placed in the
proximal end of the colon, which is then returned to the abdominal cavity. A
modified Allis clamp (Ethicon Endosurgery Inc.) is used to grasp the anvil while a
circular stapler is inserted transanally. The anvil receptacle is deployed through
the rectal stump staple line piercing the rectal wall. To allow the two ends of the
colon to be approximated it is helpful at this time to change the position of the
laparoscope to the right lower port to confirm proper orientation, lack of tension,
and exclusion of extraneous tissue prior to effecting the end-to-end anastomosis.
The procedure is concluded after assessing anastomotic integrity by transanal air
insufflation while the pelvis is filled with saline. During testing, the segment of
colon proximal to the anastomosis is occluded with an atraumatic bowel clamp.
Finally the tissue rings are inspected for completeness. An incomplete anastomosis may be repaired by laparoscopic suturing or hernia clip application,[50] redone
or, by conversion to laparotomy if necessary.

Laparoscopic Abdominoperineal Resection

Laparoscopic proctectomy is a technically feasible alternative for both cancer and
colitis[50] and may theoretically allow a more precise assessment of excision
margins.[51]

After pneumoperitoneum is established via the umbilical insertion site, the
second and third 10/12-mm trocars are placed in the right iliac fossa and right
paraumbilical regions. An additional 10/12-mm trocar is positioned in the lower
left quadrant at the site premarked for the stoma.

The rectosigmoid is mobilised and the left ureter is identified. An endoscopic
30-mm linear cutting stapler device is used to transect the inferior mesenteric
vessels and the superior haemorrhoidals. The dissection is completed with
mobilisation of the rectum in the presacral plane with identification and preservation of the pelvic sympathetic nerves. The lateral stalks are usually divided
using the harmonic scalpel (Ethicon Endosurgery Inc.). At this point perineal
dissection is performed in the standard fashion and the specimen is retrieved.
Creation of an end colostomy and closure of the perineal wound concludes the
procedure.[10]

Laparoscopic Total Abdominal Colectomy

Laparoscopic total abdominal colectomy with ileoproctostomy and laparoscopic restorative proctocolectomy are both technically feasible.[53] Indications include colitis, Crohn's disease, familial adenomatous polyposis, and colonic inertia.[39] This procedure is time-consuming and has not yet reduced the length of hospitalisation compared with laparotomy.[9,53] Nevertheless, laparoscopic total abdominal colectomy may have a role in young patients in whom improved cosmesis as achieved by the laparoscopically assisted procedure is the major desired advantage.

Five 10/12-mm ports are placed, one each in the supraumbilical site, right upper and lower quadrants and left upper and lower quadrants. The incision for the specimen retrieval and the stoma site should all be considered at the time of the port placement. The specimen may be retrieved through a Pfannenstiel incision or through the stoma site, if a stoma is planned. Division of the mesentery and transection of the terminal ileum is preferably performed extracorporeally. The end ileostomy is then delivered through the premarked site and matured as described earlier in this chapter. If the procedure is an ileorectal anastomosis, it is performed in the same fashion as the colorectal anastomosis after a laparoscopic left colectomy.

Laparoscopic Right Colectomy

Indications for this procedure include colonoscopically unresectable neoplasms, terminal ileal Crohn's disease and malignancy.

The selection of port sites depends both upon the patient's body habitus and the type of resection planned. Two monitors, one on each side of the patient, are used. The surgeon generally stands on the left side, opposite the assistant.

After the initial umbilical port is placed, a second trocar is inserted into the left iliac fossa, slightly to the left of the epigastric vessels, while a third trocar is introduced at the paraumbilical position. If needed, as in obese patients, an optional fourth port is inserted in the left upper quadrant. Mobilisation of the colon is performed and the larger omental and retroperitoneal vessels encountered at the flexures are ligated with either surgical clips or divided with the harmonic scalpel (Ethicon Endosurgery Inc.). Full mobilisation from the ileum to the mid-transverse colon includes visualisation of the duodenum and the right ureter. After complete mobilisation, a 2- to 5-cm transumbilical incision is made, incorporating the incision previously made for the Veress needle. The mesenteric vascular ligation and bowel division are then undertaken as extracorporeal procedures. A side-to-side (functional end-to-end) anastomosis is created with a linear cutting stapler device. After the mesenteric defect is repaired, the colon is delivered back to the abdominal cavity and the procedure is concluded with closure of the incision and the port sites.[27]

Laparoscopic Rectopexy for Rectal Prolapse

Although rectal prolapse is a benign condition, it can be debilitating. Surgical therapy may be approached by either the transperineal or transperitoneal routes.

Accepted transabdominal procedures include rectopexy with or without sigmoid resection.[54] Perineal procedures involve either proctosigmoidectomy or a Delorme-type of resection.[55] Laparoscopic techniques may be utilised instead of the abdominal approaches and as an adjunct to the perineal approach.[56]

For laparoscopic abdominal rectopexy the rectum is completely mobilised posteriorly to the level of the levators. Then, either a sheet of Marlex mesh (C.R. Bard, Mass.) or polypropylene mesh (Surgipro Mesh; United States Surgical Corporation, Norwalk, Conn.) is stapled to the posterior rectal wall and presacral fascia on both sides of the rectum.[57] If a sigmoid resection is desired, the rectopexy should be performed either with sutures or staples.

The perineal approach for the surgical treatment of a complete rectal prolapse may be assisted by the laparoscopic technique for transabdominal mobilisation of the rectum to facilitate a more extensive perineal resection of the rectosigmoid.[58] Furthermore the laparoscope can be transperineally introduced after delivering a sufficiently long segment of prolapsed rectum. The remaining rectum, sigmoid or left colon is now visualised and further mobilisation for the resection is undertaken if necessary. The procedure is concluded with resection of the prolapsed segment and subsequent coloanal anastomosis and levatoroplasty.[33]

Laparoscopy for Intestinal Obstruction

Indications for laparoscopic adhesiolysis include patients who have had previous abdominal surgery and present with transient recurrent episodes or an acute progressive onset of intestinal obstruction.[59] This procedure allows efficient diagnosis and usually effective treatment in cases of an undetermined cause of intestine obstruction.[60,61] It should not generally be applied for the treatment of chronic abdominal pain.

The initial creation of pneumoperitoneum should be carefully planned and executed. When choosing the site for placement of the first trocar, previous incisions, including scars from previous laparoscopy, should be avoided if possible. After the site is chosen, an open technique is used to insert a blunt–tip Hasson trocar or a 10-mm port with video capability. If the initial site is amid multiple adhesions, an effort should be made to close the fascia to prevent air leakage and an alternative site should be chosen.

After the placement of the first trocar, the laparoscope is inserted, and careful inspection ensues. Quite often, visibility is limited due to adhesions, and at least one port should be inserted under direct vision before exploration is undertaken. All ports should be 10–12 mm in size to provide flexibility in camera and instrument positioning. As the adhesions are lysed and more of the peritoneal cavity inspected, additional ports are placed. Once the abdominal wall is cleared of adhesions, careful inspection of the bowel is undertaken. As it is often difficult to assess which of the adhesions were responsible for the clinical symptoms, especially in elective cases, sound judgment should be used and all adhesions which would be divided during a laparotomy should be lysed. Ideally, collapsed distal and dilated proximal bowel should be confirmed. According to the findings, additional laparoscopic or laparoscopic-assisted procedures such as bowel resection, anastomosis, hernia reduction and repair, or stoma creation is performed.[61]

Laparoscopic Surgery for Colorectal Malignancy

Several concerns have arisen regarding adequate laparoscopic excision of a neoplasm, especially for rectal cancer where the surgical technique plays a critical role in the prevention of local recurrence. In the case of rectal cancer, it has been demonstrated that an incomplete surgical excision of the mesorectum and an inadequate lateral margin clearance[62–66] are both associated with increased locoregional failure and poor prognosis. An improved 5-year survival rate of 78% and local recurrence of 3–5% has been achieved by Heald et al.[67] by routine total mesorectal excision. More recently others have confirmed Heald's results.[68–71]

Recent experience indicates that complete mesorectal excision with wide lateral margins is easily done through the laparoscope.[12,72,73] The rectum, after full mobilisation, can be retracted in a cephalad direction, thus facilitating the dissection in the avascular presacral space. Any advantage of radical abdominopelvic lymphadenectomy for rectal cancer, as advocated by several authors[74,75] still needs to be determined.[76] There are only a few experimental reports in the literature of such a lymphatic excision by laparoscopy.[77,78]

Some authors consider high ligation of inferior mesenteric artery and harvesting of a large number of lymph nodes to be part of a curative resection for colonic neoplasm with improving survival rates.[79,80] This issue remains controversial and some studies have failed to demonstrate any advantages for patients treated by high ligation of the inferior mesenteric artery.[81,82]

Many recent studies have failed to demonstrate any significant differences between the numbers of lymph nodes removed when comparing laparoscopy and laparotomy.[83–85] The absolute number of lymph nodes laparoscopically removed cannot be taken as a criterion for the effectiveness of a surgical excision, because the number of lymph nodes collected depends not only on the surgeon, but also on the enthusiasm and technique of lymph node isolation employed by the pathologist.[86,87]

A critical issue related to laparoscopic surgery for cancer is the problem of port site tumour recurrence (wound implantation) Since Alexander et al.[88] first reported a 67-year-old female patient with a wound recurrence after laparoscopic-assisted right hemicolectomy for a Dukes' A carcinoma, many port site recurrences following laparoscopic procedures for cure of malignancy have been described.[89] This complication has occurred not only in the port site through which the specimen is delivered, but has involved all port sites. While most port site recurrences occur in the setting of advanced disease and carcinomatosis, a significant number have been found after curative resection for relatively early disease.[90] In fact, these phenomena have occurred following laparoscopic cholecystectomy for an unsuspected occult gall bladder carcinoma[88,91] and after laparoscopic appendectomy in a patient with an occult carcinoma. It has certainly occurred many times in patients with early stage colon carcinomas. The aetiology remains controversial, yet there are experimental data suggesting that surgical wounds are fertile sites for neoplastic growth.[92,93]

The fact that this complication is virtually absent after laparotomy[94,95] suggests that pneumoperitoneum may play an important role in its development.[96] The actual incidence of port site recurrence is unknown. Vertruyen et al.[97] noted an overall 3.5% incidence. Similar numbers were found by other authors.[98–102] At opposite ends of the spectrum, Berends et al.[103] and Molenaar et al.[104] reported incidences of 14% and 21%, respectively, and Ramos et al.[105],

Vukasin et al.[106] and Fleshman et al.[107] demonstrated a 1–1.5% incidence of port site recurrence. Putting the problem in perspective, isolated wound implantation without peritoneal carcinomatosis occurs after laparotomy in between 0.1% and 0.3% of cases.[94,95] In the series reported by Ramos[108] the incidence of port site recurrence in the absence of peritoneal carcinomatosis was as low as 0.48%. The denominator may be increasing as a recent study showed that 4.6% of members of the American Society of Colon and Rectal Surgeons and Society of American Gastrointestinal Endoscopic Surgeons have seen port site recurrence.[109]

Laparoscopic resections for cure of carcinoma are still highly controversial and are by no means a standard of care. In light of this controversy, prospective, randomised controlled trials have been undertaken in at least six countries[110] to address this question. Unfortunately, conclusions will not be available for at least 5 years. The consensus is that laparoscopic resection of colorectal carcinoma should be limited to use in prospective randomised externally monitored trials. However, palliation of metastatic disease may be a good laparoscopic indication.

Developing Laparoscopic Expertise

Before embarking on laparoscopic colorectal surgery the surgeon should be comfortable with all facets of diagnosis and treatment of colorectal pathology in the traditional manner.[111] Next the surgeon must obtain basic laparoscopic skills. For those surgeons currently in training this goal has been incorporated into the surgical residency curriculum.[112,113] However, for the majority of surgeons who have already completed residency training, attendance at a course to obtain this advanced training is required.[90]

The learning curve of laparoscopic colorectal procedures is associated with longer operative times and increased intraoperative complication rates.[12,98,114] With more experience and improved technology, these problems can be overcome.[115] Agachan et al.[116] demonstrated a significant decrease in mean operative time suggesting that the learning curve plateaus after 70 cases. However, the same conclusion can be reached by a significant decrease in intraoperative complications after 55 procedures. Change in the learning curve also reflects a change in case selection as noted by Agachan et al.[115]

Conclusion

Laparoscopic colorectal surgery has been well established as more complex and larger surgical procedures have been safely and successfully performed.

Although laparoscopic surgery for the treatment of benign colorectal disorders is readily accepted, this same technique for the management of malignancy has yet to be proven better or even as efficacious as laparotomy. Distant and local recurrences, long-term survival and port site recurrences are still issues to be better clarified through controlled, prospective, randomised trials.

References

1. Dubois F, Icard P, Berthelot G, Levard H (1990) Coeliscopic cholecystectomy. Preliminary report of 36 cases. Ann Surg 211:60–62.
2. Reddick EJ, Olsen DO (1989) Laparoscopic laser cholecystectomy: a comparison with mini-laparotomy cholecystectomy. Surg Endosc 3:131–133.
3. Cuschieri A, Berci G, McSherry CK (1990) Laparoscopic cholecystectomy. Am J Surg 159:273–278.
4. DeKok H (1977) A new technique for resecting the noninflamed not-adhesive appendix through a mini-laparotomy with the aid of a laparoscope. Arch Chir Neerl 29:195.
5. Semm K (1983) Endoscopic appendectomy. Endoscopy 15:59–64.
6. Schreiber JH (1987) Early experience with laparoscopic appendectomy in women. Surg Endosc 1:211–216.
7. Whitworth CM, Whitworth PW, Sanfillipo J, Polk HC Jr. (1988) Value of diagnostic laparoscopy in young women with possible appendicitis. Surg Gynecol Obstet 167:187–190.
8. Monson JRT, Darzi A, Carey PD, Guillou PJ (1992) Prospective evaluation of laparoscopic-assisted colectomy in an unselected group of patients. Lancet 340:831–833.
9. Schmitt SL, Cohen SM, Wexner SD, Nogueras JJ, Jagelman DG (1994) Does laparoscopic-assisted ileal pouch anal anastomosis reduce the length of hospitalization? Int J Colorectal Dis 9:134–137.
10. Larach SW, Salomon MC, Williamson PR, Goldstein E (1993) Laparoscopic-assisted abdominoperineal resection. Surg Laparosc Endosc 3:115–118.
11. Tate JJT, Kwok S, Dawson JW, Lau WY, Li AK (1993) Prospective comparison of laparoscopic and conventional anterior resection. Br J Surg 80:1396–1398.
12. Guillou OJ, Darzi A, Monson JR (1993) Experience with laparoscopic colorectal surgery for malignant disease. Surg Oncol 2(Suppl 1):43–49.
13. Wexner SD, Cohen SM, Johansen OB, Nogueras JJ, Jagelman DG (1993) Laparoscopic colorectal surgery: a prospective assessment and current perspective. Br J Surg 80:1602–1605.
14. Pfeifer J, Wexner SD, Reissman P, Bernstein M, Nogueras JJ, Singh S, Weiss EG (1995) Laparoscopy versus open colon surgery: costs and outcome. Surg Endosc 9:1322–1326.
15. Jacobs M, Verdeja JC, Goldstein HS (1991) Minimally invasive colon resection (laparoscopic colectomy) Surg Laparosc Endosc 1:144–150.
16. Franklin MEJr, Ramos R, Rosenthal D, Schuessler W (1993) Laparoscopic colonic procedures. World J Surg 17:51–56.
17. Jenkins DM, Paluzzi M, Scott TE (1993) Postlaparoscopic small bowel obstruction. Surg Laparosc Endosc 3:139–141.
18. Phillips EH, Franklin M, Carroll BJ, Fallas MJ, Ramos R, Rosenthal D (1992) Laparoscopic colectomy. Ann Surg 216:703–707.
19. Chen HH, Alabaz O, Iroatulam AJN, Nessim A, Joo JS, Weiss EG, Nogueras JJ, Wexner SD (1997) Laparoscopic colectomy for benign colorectal disease is associated with a significant reduction in disability as compared to laparotomy. Surg Endosc 12:1397–1400.
20. Böhm B, Milsom JW, Fazio VW (1995) Postoperative intestinal motility following conventional and laparoscopic intestinal surgery. Arch Surg 130:415–419.
21. Binderow SR, Cohen SM, Wexner SD, Nogueras JJ (1994) Must early postoperative oral intake be limited to laparoscopy? Dis Colon Rectum 37:584–589.
22. Reissman P, Teoh TA, Weiss EG, Cohen SM, Nogueras JJ, Wexner SD (1995) Is early feeding safe after elective colorectal surgery? Ann Surg 222:73–77.
23. Ramos JM, Beart RW, Goes R, Ortega AE, Schlinkert RT (1995) Role of laparoscopy in colorectal surgery. A prospective evaluation of 200 cases. Dis Colon Rectum 38:494–501.
24. Reiver D, Kmiot WA, Cohen SM, Weiss EG, Nogueras JJ, Wexner SD (1994) A prospective comparison of laparoscopic procedures in colorectal surgery. Dis Colon Rectum 37:22 (abstract).
25. Falk PM, Beart RW, Wexner SD, Thorson AG, Jagelman DG, Lavery IC, Johansen OB, Fitzgibbons RJ Jr (1993) Laparoscopic colectomy: a critical appraisal. Dis Colon Rectum 36:28–34.
26. Senagore AJ, Luchtefeld MA, Mackeigan JM, Mazier WP (1993) Open colectomy versus laparoscopic colectomy: are there differences? Am Surg 59:549–554.
27. Cohen SM, Wexner SD (1994) Laparoscopic right hemicolectomy. Surg Rounds: Min Invasive Surg 627–635.
28. Fleshman JW, Fry PD, Birnbaum EH, Kodner IJ (1996) Laparoscopic assisted and minilaparotomy approaches to colorectal diseases are similar in early outcome. Dis Colon Rectum 39:15–22.

29. Lazorthes F, Chiotassol P (1986) Stapled colorectal anastomosis: perspective integrity of the anastomosis and risk of postoperative leakage. Int J Colorectal Dis 1:96–98.
30. Wexner SD, Beck DE (1993) Sepsis prevention in colorectal surgery. In: Fielding LP, Goldberg SM (eds) Operative surgery of the colon, rectum and anus, 5th edn. Butterworth, London, pp 41–46.
31. Oliveira L, Wexner SD, Daniel N, DeMarta D, Weiss EG, Nogueras JJ, Bernstein M. (1997) Mechanical bowel preparation for elective colorectal surgery. A prospective, randomized, surgeon-blinded trial comparing sodium phosphate and polyethylene glycol based oral lavage solutions. Dis Colon Rectum 40:585–591.
32. Hasson HM (1971) Modified instrument and method for laparoscopy. Am J Obstet Gynecol 110: 886–887.
33. Reissman P, Weiss EG, Teoh TA, Cohen SM, Wexner SD (1995) Laparoscopic assisted perineal rectosigmoidectomy for rectal prolapse. Surg Laparosc Endosc 5: 217–218.
34. Nogueras JJ, Wexner SD (1992) Laparoscopic colon resection. Perspec Colon Rectal Surg 5:79–97.
35. Corbitt JD Jr (1992) Preliminary experience with laparoscopic-guided colectomy. Surg Laparosc Endosc 2:79–81.
36. Larach SW, Salomon MC, Williamson PR, Goldstein E (1993) Laparoscopic-assisted colectomy: experience during the learning curve. Coloproctology 1: 38–41.
37. Wexner SD, Cohen SM, Ulrich A, Reissman P (1995) Laparoscopic colorectal surgery: are we being honest with our patients? Dis Colon Rectum 38: 723–727.
38. Teoh, TA, Wexner SD (1996) Laparoscopic surgery in colorectal cancer. In Williams NS (ed) Colorectal cancer. Churchill Livingstone, Edinburgh.
39. Bernstein MA, Dawson JW, Reissman P, Weiss EG, Nogueras JJ, Wexner SD (1996) Is complete laparoscopic colectomy superior to laparoscopic-assisted colectomy? Am Surg 62: 507–511
40. Knight CD, Griffen FD (1980) An improved technique for low anterior resection of the rectum using the EEA stapler. Surgery 88:710–714.
41. Oliveira L, Reissman P, Nogueras J, Wexner SD (1997) Laparoscopic creation of stomas. Surg Endosc 11: 19–23.
42. Wexner SD, Gonzalez-Padron A, Teoh TA, Moon HK (1996) The stimulated gracilis neosphincter for fecal incontinence: a new use for an old concept. Plast Reconstruct Surg 98:693–699.
43. Romero CA, James KM, Cooperstone LM, Mishrick AS, Ger R (1992) Laparoscopic sigmoid colostomy for perineal Crohn's disease. Surg Laparosc Endosc 2:148–151.
44. Fuhrman G, Ota DM (1994) Laparoscopic intestinal stomas. Dis Colon Rectum 37:444–449.
45. Lange V, Meyer G, Shardey M, Schildberg FW (1991) Laparoscopic creation of a loop ileostomy. J Laparoendosc Surg 1:307–312.
46. Khoo RE, Montrey J, Cohen MM (1993) Laparoscopic loop ileostomy for temporary fecal diversion. Dis Colon Rectum 36:966–968.
47. Teoh TA, Reissman P, Cohen SM, Weiss EG, Wexner SD (1994) Laparoscopic loop ileostomy. Dis Colon Rectum 37:514 (letter).
48. Pier A, Gotz F, Bacher C (1991) Laparoscopic appendectomy in 625 cases: from innovation to routine. Surg Laparosc Endosc 1:8–13.
49. Wexner SD, Cohen SM (1996) Laparoscopic appendectomy and colectomy. In: Zuidema GD (ed). Surgery of the alimentary tract, 4th edn. Saunders, Philadelphia.
50. Cohen SM, Clem MF, Wexner SD, Jagelman DG (1994) An initial comparative study of two techniques of laparoscopic colonic anastomosis and mesenteric defect closure. Surg Endosc 8:130–134
51. Wu JS, Birnbaum EH (1997) Early experience with laparoscopic abdominoperineal resection. Surg Endosc 11:449–455.
52. Darzi A, Lewis C, Menzies–Gow N, Guillou PJ, Monson JR (1995) Laparoscopic abdominoperineal excision of the rectum. Surg Endosc 9:414–417.
53. Wexner SD, Johansen OB, Nogueras JJ, Jagelman DG (1992) Laparoscopic total abdominal colectomy. A prospective trial. Dis Colon Rectum 35:651–655.
54. Rhodes M, Stitz RW (1994) Laparoscopic subtotal colectomy. Semin Colon Rectal Surg 5:267–270.
55. Keighley MR, Fielding JW, Alexander-Williams J (1983) Results of marlex mesh abdominal rectopexy for rectal prolapse in 100 consecutive patients. Br J Surg 70:229–232.
56. Altemeier WA, Culbertson WR, Schowengerdt C, Hunt J (1971) Nineteen years experience with the one-stage perineal repair of rectal prolapse. Ann Surg 173:993–1006.
57. Cuschieri A, Shimi SM, Vander Velpen G, Banting S, Wood RA (1994) Laparoscopic prosthesis fixation rectopexy for complete rectal prolapse. Br J Surg 8:138–139.
58. Darzi A, Henry MM, Guillou PJ, Shorvon P, Monson JR (1995) Stapled laparoscopic rectopexy for rectal prolapse. Surg Endosc 9:301–303.

59. Lointier P, Lechner C, Larpent J L, Chipponi J (1993) Laparoscopic assisted perineal rectosigmoidectomy with pullthrough. J Laparoendosc Surg 3:547–556.

60. Silva PD, Cogbill TH (1991) Laparoscopic treatment of recurrent small bowel obstruction. Wis Med J 90:169–170.

61. François Y, Mouret P, Tomaoglu K, Vignal J (1994) Postoperative adhesive peritoneal disease: laparoscopic treatment. Surg Endosc 8:781–783.

62. Reissman P, Wexner SD (1995) Laparoscopic surgery for intestinal obstruction. Surg Endosc 9:865–868.

63. Cooperman A, Katz V, Zimmon D, Botero G (1991) Laparoscopic colon resection: a case report. J Laparoendosc Surg 1:221–224.

64. Heald RJ, Husband E, Ryall RD (1982) The mesorectum in rectal cancer surgery: the clue to pelvic recurrence. Br J Surg 69:613–616.

65. Ng I O, Luk IS, Yuen ST, Lau PW, Pritchett CJ, Ng M, Poon GP, Ho J (1993) Surgical lateral clearance in resected rectal carcinomas: a multivariate analysis of clinicopathologic features. Cancer 71:1972–1976.

66. Quirke P, Durdey P, Dixon MF, Williams NS (1986) Local recurrence of rectal adenocarcinoma due to inadequate surgical resection. Lancet I:996–999.

67. Heald RJ, Ryall RD (1986) Recurrence and survival after total mesorectal excision for rectal cancer. Lancet I:1479–1482.

68. Enker WE, Thaler HT, Cranor ML, Polyak T (1995) Total mesorectal excision in the operative treatment of carcinoma of the rectum. J Am Coll Surg 181:335–346.

69. Arbman G, Nilsson E, Hallbook O, Sjodahl R (1996) Local recurrence following total mesorectal excision for rectal cancer. Br J Surg 83:375–379.

70. Scott N, Jackson P, al-Jaberi T, Dixon MF, Quirke P, Finan PJ (1995) Total mesorectal excision and local recurrence: a study of tumor spread in the mesorectum distal to rectal cancer. Br J Surg 82:1031–1033.

71. Aitken RJ (1996) Mesorectal excision for rectal cancer. Br J Surg 83:214–216.

72. Bernstein MA, Bin A, Weiss EG, Nogueras JJ, Wexner SD (1998) Total mesorectal excision without adjuvant therapy for local control of rectal cancer: a North American experience. Techniques in Coloproctology 2:11–15.

73. Iroatulam AJ, Agachan F, Alabaz O, Weiss EG, Nogueras JJ, Wexner SD (1998) Laparoscopic abdomino perineal resection for anorectal cancer. Am Surg 64:12–18.

74. Leung KL, Kwok SP, Lau WY, Meng WC, Lam TY, Kwong KH, Chung CC, Li AK (1997) Laparoscopic-assisted resection of rectosigmoid carcinoma. Immediate and medium-term results. Arch Surg 132:761–764.

75. Enker W, Laffer VT, Block GE (1979) Enhanced survival of patients with colon and rectal cancer is based upon wide anatomic resection. Ann Surg 190:350–360.

76. Koyama Y, Moriya Y, Hojo K (1984) Effects of extended systemic lymphadenectomy for adenocarcinoma of the rectum: significant improvement of survival rate and decrease of local recurrence. Jpn J Clin Oncol 14:131–632.

77. Harnsberger JR, Vernava AM III, Longo WE (1994) Radical abdominopelvic lymphadenectomy: historic perspective and current role in the surgical management of rectal cancer. Dis Colon Rectum 37:73–87.

78. Decanini C, Milsom JW, Bohm B, Fazio VW (1994) Laparoscopic oncologic abdominoperineal resection. Dis Colon Rectum 37:552–558.

79. Karamura YJ, Savada T, Muto T, Nagai H (1994) Laparoscopic assisted colectomy and lymphadenectomy with abdominal wall lifting method. Dis Colon Rectum 37:16.

80. Bacon HE, Khubchandani IT (1964) The rationale of aortoileopelvic and high ligation of the inferior mesenteric artery for carcinoma of the left half of the colon and rectum. Surg Gynecol Obstet 119:503–508.

81. Sugarbaker PH, Corlew S (1982) Influence of surgical technique on survival in patients with colorectal cancer: a review. Dis Colon Rectum 25:545–557.

82. Grinnel RS (1965) Results of ligation of inferior mesenteric artery at the aorta in resections of carcinoma of the descending sigmoid and colon and rectum. Surg Gynecol Obstet 120:1031–1036.

83. Pezim ME, Nicholls RJ (1984) Survival after high or low ligation of the inferior mesenteric artery during curative surgery of rectal cancer. Ann Surg 200:729–733.

84. Kim HJ, Roy T (1994) Unexpected gallbladder cancer with cutaneous seeding after laparoscopic cholecystectomy. South Med J 87:817–820.

85. Franklin ME Jr, Rosenthal D, Norem RF (1995) Prospective evaluation of laparoscopic colon resection versus open colon resection for adenocarcinoma. A multicenter study. Surg Endosc 9:811–816.

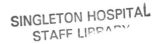

86.   Lord SA, Larach SW, Ferrara A, Williamson PR, Lago CP, Lube MW (1996) Laparoscopic resections for colorectal carcinoma. A three-year experience. Dis Colon Rectum 39:148-154.
87.   Cohen SM, Wexner SD, Schmitt SL, Nogueras JJ, Lucas FV (1994) Effect of xylene clearance of mesenteric fat on harvest of lymph nodes after colonic resection. Eur J Surg 160:693-697.
88.   Alexander RJ, Jacques BC, Mitchell KG (1993) Laparoscopically assisted colectomy and wound recurrence. Lancet 341:249-250 (letter).
89.   Nduka CC, Monson JRT, Menzies-Gown, Darzi A (1994) Abdominal wall metastases following laparoscopy. Br J Surg 81:648-652.
90.   Wexner SD, Cohen SM (1995) Port site metastases after laparoscopic surgery for cure of malignancy: a plea for caution. Br J Surg 82:295-298.
91.   Weiss EG, Wexner SD (1996) Laparoscopic port site recurrence in oncologic surgery. a review. Ann Acad Med Singapore 25:694-698.
92.   Clair DG, Lautz DB, Brooks DC (1993) Rapid development of umbilical metastases after cholecystectomy for unsuspected gallbladder carcinoma. Surgery 113:355-358.
93.   Murthy SM, Goldschmidt RA, Rhao LN, Ammirati M, Buchmann T, Scanlon EF (1989) The influence of surgical trauma on experimental metastases. Cancer 64:2035-2044.
94.   Hughes ES, McDermott FT, Polglase AL, Johnson WR (1983) Tumor recurrence in the abdominal wall scar after large bowel cancer surgery. Dis Colon Rectum 26:571-572.
95.   Reilly WT, Nelson H, Schroeder G, Wieand HS, Bolton J, O'Connell MJ (1996) Wound recurrence following conventional treatment of colorectal cancer. A rare but perhaps underestimated problem. Dis Colon Rectum 39:200-207.
96.   Whelan RL, Sellers GJ, Allendorf JD, Laird D, Bessler MD, Nowygrod R, Treat MR (1996) Trocar site recurrence is unlikely to result from aerosolization of tumor cells. Dis Colon Rectum 39(Suppl):7-13.
97.   Vertruyen M, Cadiere GB, Himpens J, Bruyn SJ, Lemper JC, Urbain D (1996) Laparosocpic colectomy for cancer. Surg Endosc 10:558 (abstract).
98.   Ngoi SS, Kum CK, Goh PMY et al. (1993) Laparoscopic colon resection: the Singapore experience. Poster presentation (P56) at the Tripartite Colorectal meeting. Sydney, Australia.
99.   Prasad A, Avery C, Foley RJG (1994) Abdominal wall metastases following laparoscopy. Br J Surg 81:1697 (letter).
100. Boulez J, Herriot E (1994) Multicentric analysis of laparoscopic colorectal surgery in FDCL group: 274 cases. Br J Surg 81:527.
101. Fingerhut A (1996) Laparoscopic-assisted colonic resection: the French experience. In: Jager R, Wexner SD (eds) Laparoscopic colorectal surgery. Churchill Livingstone, New York, pp 253-257.
102. Molenaar CB, Bijnen AB, Ruiter P (1998) Indications for laparoscopic colorectal surgery. Surg Endosc 12:42-45.
103. Berends FJ, Lange JF, Bonjer HJ, Kazemier G (1994) Subcutaneous metastases after laparoscopic colectomy. Lancet 344:58
104. Molenaar CBH, Bijnen AB, Lopes-Cardozo AMF, de Ruiter P (1996) Indications for laparoscopic colectomy. Presented at the XVIth Biennial Congress of the International Society of University Colon and Rectal Surgeons. Lisbon, Portugal, 14-18 April 1996.
105. Ramos JM, Gupta S, Anthone GJ, Ortega AE, Simons AJ, Beart RW (1994) Laparoscopic colon cancer: is the port site at risk? A preliminary report. Arch Surg 129:897-900.
106. Vukasin P, Ortega AE, Greene FL, Steele GD, Simons AJ, Anthone GJ, Weston LA, Beart RW (1996) Wound recurrence following laparoscopic colon resection: results of the American Society of Colon and Rectal Surgeons Laparoscopic Registry. Dis Colon Rectum 39(Suppl):S20-S23.
107. Fleshman JW, Nelson H, Peters WR et al., Clinical Outcomes of Surgical Therapy (COST) Study Group (1996) Early results of laparoscopic surgery for colorectal cancer: retrospective analysis of 372 patients treated by COST Study Group. Dis Colon Rectum 39(Suppl):S53-S58.
108. Ramos R (1994) Complications in laparoscopic colon surgery: prevention and management. Semin Colon Rectal Surg 5:239.
109. Mavrantonis C, Potenti F, Wexner SD (1998) Laparoscopic colorectal surgery: have attitudes changed? Dis Colon Rectum 41:A47 (abstract).
110. Sackier JM, Wexner SD (eds) (1998) Protocols in general surgery laparoscopic colorectal surgery. Wiley, New York.
111. Cuschieri A (1992) The dust has settled – let's sweep it clean: training in minimal access surgery. J R Coll Surg Edinb 37:213-214 (editorial).
112. Bailey RW, Imbembo AL, Zucker KA (1991) Establishment of laparoscopic cholecystectomy training program. Am Surg 57:231-236.

113. Laws HI (1991) Credentialing residents for laparoscopic surgery: a matter of opinion. Curr Surg 684.
114. Fingerhut A (1994) Laparoscopic colorectal surgery. Presented at the World Congress of Endoscopic Surgery, Kyoto, Japan.
115. Agachan F, Gilliland R, Joo JS, Sher ME, Wexner SD (1996) The impact of experience on the outcome of laparoscopic colorectal surgery over four years. Surg Endosc 10:219 (abstract).
116. Agachan F, Joo JS, Weiss EG, Wexner SD (1996) Intraoperative laparoscopic complications. Are we getting better? Dis Colon Rectal 514–519.

3 Combined Surgical Treatment for Advanced Pelvic Malignancy

N.D. Carr and M.G. Lucas

Introduction

Total pelvic exenteration or one of its modifications may seem a daunting prospect for both surgeon and patient alike. However, there is no doubt that a great deal can be achieved by the removal of these advanced primary or recurrent tumours and related structures in terms of achieving maximum palliation or even cure.[1-6] Although adjuvant treatment with radiotherapy, chemotherapy or both of these modalities may also be required, there is controversy about their value[7] and the principle of surgical removal of all or most of the tumour bulk should be foremost in the clinician's mind.[2,5]

Whilst there are those who advocate that a single "superspecialist" should undertake these operations, the present authors believe that a multidisciplinary approach is to be preferred. We do not support the concept of the gynaecological oncologist who aims to be a "total pelvic surgeon". It is unlikely that any one individual can acquire the wide range of skills necessary to perform radical gynaecological, colorectal and urological surgery as well as the appropriate reconstructive techniques. Moreover, the expertise of a plastic surgeon is often required. Even in large centres it is unlikely that more than a few of these operations would be performed in a year and so there is a strong argument for centralising these operations to places where a multidisciplinary team and all of the necessary backup facilities exist.[8] A multidisciplinary approach to these complex surgical problems not only offers the patient the best standard of care for each aspect of the surgery, but will encourage a sharing of knowledge and skills that can only enhance the abilities of the entire team.

The purpose of this chapter is to consider the indications for, the surgical principles of, and the outcome of radical surgery for primary and recurrent pelvic malignancy.

Indications for and the Principles of Surgery

Types of Pelvic Exenteration

Total pelvic exenteration (TPE) for the treatment of advanced pelvic malignancy was first reported by Brunschwig in 1948.[9] Over the next 15 years others reported similar experience,[10-13] whilst the past 15 years have witnessed numerous authors reporting large retrospective series of TPE or one of its modifications in the surgical management of advanced or recurrent carcinoma of the cervix, ovary, vagina, uterus,[14,15] sigmoid colon and rectum,[16-18] bladder,[19] prostate[20] and other organs.[21-23]

Although original descriptions of this operation involved removal of the entire pelvic viscera with both urinary and faecal diversion, excision may be limited to the anterior or posterior pelvis. For example anterior pelvic exenteration (APE) implies removal of the bladder, distal ureters, reproductive organs in the female and pelvic peritoneum and may be indicated when the rectum is not involved by tumour. By contrast, posterior pelvic exenteration (PPE) spares the bladder and distal ureters but involves excision of the rectum, sigmoid colon, reproductive organs in the female and pelvic peritoneum (Fig. 3.1).

It is also helpful to consider the resection in terms of its relationship to the pelvic floor in that resection may be supralevator, infralevator or involve excision of the perineal tissues. Some surgical decisions can only be made at the time of operation and hence surgical versatility is important. Moreover, all members of the team should perform ablative and reconstructive pelvic surgery regularly within their own field. These cases are not for the generalist.

Indications for Radical Excision

There are certain tumours which may be suitable for the consideration of radical resection (Table 3.1), and although this series by Lopez et al.[18] provides

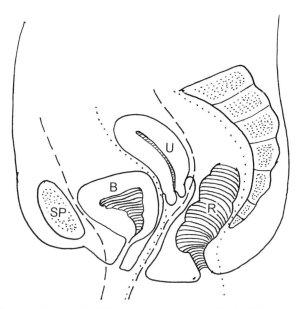

Fig. 3.1. Sagittal section showing the difference between anterior (dashed line) and posterior (dotted line) pelvic exenterations. Total pelvic exenteration lies between anterior dashed line and posterior dotted line. SP, symphysis pubis; B, bladder; U, uterus ; R, rectum.

Table 3.1. Tumours which are suitable for radical excision

Site	n (%)
Cervix	155 (67)
Rectum	27 (12)
Endometrium	16 (7)
Vagina	9 (4)
Bladder	5 (2)
Ovary	5 (2)
Anus	4 (1.7)
Vulva	4 (1.7)
Urethra	2 (0.8)
Prostate	2 (0.8)
Pelvic sarcoma	2 (0.8)
Skin	1 (0.4)
Total	232 (100)

From Lopez et al.[18]

an excellent background upon which to base current indications, it should now be realized that most carcinomas of the cervix are primarily treated by radiotherapy. Conversely, many locally advanced rectal cancers that, hitherto, would have been managed by non-invasive methods are now being seriously considered for radical resection.[17,23] Radical pelvic surgery may also be required for patients who have sustained the severe complications of pelvic radiotherapy such as fistulae, obstruction and hypocompliance of the urinary and colorectal systems.[7]

Aims of Surgery

The aims of surgery can be either curative or palliative. Curative surgery will require eradication of all demonstrable disease from the pelvis whatever the extent of exenteration involved. This may involve removal of the rectum, bladder and entire perineum. Retrorectal sarcomas and other tumours which have invaded the lower sacrum may require removal of part of the sacrum as well.[23–25] Vascular reconstruction should also be considered in those tumours that have invaded major vessels at the pelvic brim and where excision of them allows potentially curative resection of the tumour. There are many permutations and combinations of what can be done and often considerable surgical ingenuity is required.

The justification for palliative resection is that subsequent radiotherapy or chemotherapy may then adequately control residual disease. Perhaps the best example of this is provided by "cytoreductive debulking" of ovarian tumours in which various intra-abdominal organs in addition to pelvic ones may require removal. Some maturity of judgement is required in these circumstances to balance the pursuit of cancer clearance against the probable morbidity of extensive resectional surgery. In addition, palliative surgery is often justified to help to control the inevitable symptoms of discharge, pain, strangury, tenesmus and leakage of urine or faeces, which are the result of advanced cancer of either the urinary or colorectal systems.[26]

Preoperative Considerations

Preoperative Staging

Patients with advanced pelvic tumours require careful preoperative imaging using standard or spiral computed tomography (CT), magnetic resonance imaging (MRI), endorectal ultrasound and transvaginal ultrasound in order to assess the degree of local spread and the presence or absence of liver metastases (Figs. 3.2, 3.3). Examination under anaesthesia by the surgical team should always be performed and provides direct evidence of tumour fixity to adjacent organs, the pelvic floor, the pelvic sidewalls and the bony sacrum. It is only by performing these investigations that the surgical team can anticipate the extent of resection and methods of reconstruction that will be required. Conversely, there is no point in subjecting a patient with advanced pelvic malignancy to laparotomy only to find that the lesion is locally inoperable. The assessment of lymph node status by laparoscopy and fine needle biopsy, whilst theoretically desirable, does not influence the team's decision to undertake aggressive resection when the aim of surgery becomes the maximal palliation of symptoms rather than potential cure. It should also be remembered that previous pelvic radiotherapy may produce fibrosis and induration of pelvic organs, apparent both on imaging and at surgical exploration, which may be indistinguishable from malignant invasion.

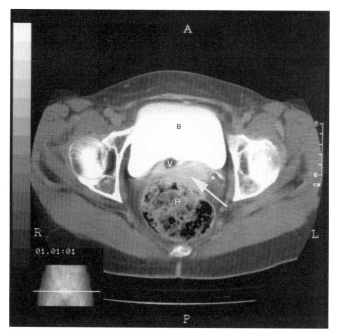

Fig. 3.2. Computed tomography (CT) scan showing a recurrent deposit of ovarian cancer (white arrow) invading the bladder (B) anteriorly, the vagina (V) and the rectum (R) posteriorly. Composite excision of these organs was necessary in this case.

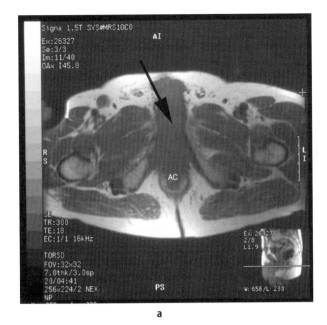

a

b

Fig. 3.3. Magnetic resonance (MR) scan in transverse section (**a**) and sagittal section (**b**) of an extensive urethral carcinoma (black arrow) which had invaded the rectum (R), the bladder base (B) and the soft tissues of the perineum. SP, symphysis pubis.

Communication

Multidisciplinary surgery requires careful preoperative planning in order to ensure that the ablative and reconstructive issues involved are understood by all the surgeons involved. An often overlooked aspect of preoperative preparation of the patient is careful counselling by the relevant subspecialist nurses, who can discuss the various options available. For example, there is no point in performing major and complicated reconstructions of the rectum and bladder in a patient who would be quite happy with a faecal and urinary diversion. Furthermore, information can be provided concerning postoperative sexual, bowel and urinary function.[27]

Anatomical Considerations

The goal of the surgery of advanced pelvic malignancy is total ablation of the disease or maximal palliation by excising most of the lesion and involved organs. Preoperatively, it should be decided whether it will be possible to preserve the anal sphincter mechanism, the urethral sphincter, the pelvic floor, the perineum, the bladder and prostate, all or part of the rectum, the vagina and the coccyx and lower sacrum. Nevertheless, reconstruction with restoration of optimal sexual, bowel and urinary function, although desirable, is a secondary consideration. Furthermore, many patients with advanced pelvic tumours are in poor medical and nutritional condition and there is a certain virtue in performing the quickest and least complicated procedure that is likely to be complicated by a low postoperative morbidity and mortality. These patients are often best served by urinary and faecal diversion.

Previous Pathology

A history of inflammatory bowel disease (IBD) or pelvic radiotherapy may influence surgical management of advanced pelvic tumours. For example, it is unwise to preserve the colon in patients who have established ulcerative or Crohn's colitis when an ileostomy may be preferable to a colostomy. If reconstruction is undertaken then it may be better to perform an ileoanal pouch rather than colorectal anastomosis. Similarly, in patients with a previous history of Crohn's disease, careful "mapping" of small bowel disease is essential.

Those patients who have received previous pelvic radiotherapy present special problems. Dissection planes may be obscured, the distal small bowel may not be suitable for either anastomosis or an ileal conduit, there may be ureteric stenosis that will make ureteric re-implantation difficult and there may be subclinical anal sphincter injury that may deem low colorectal anastomosis unwise. Clearly, these factors will have to be considered by the surgical team and appropriate alterations in strategy made.

Anaesthesia and Postoperative Care

Although pelvic exenteration has been employed for over 40 years[1] there is no doubt that one of the major contributors to improved outcome has been the advance of anaesthesia and high-dependency postoperative care. Thromboembolic prophylaxis, careful fluid and electrolyte management and hyperalimentation are all essential for these patients. Autologous blood salvage has reduced the need for donor transfusion and epidural anaesthesia for postoperative pain relief is a major benefit. These procedures should not be done without experienced anaesthetists and the availability of high-dependency or intensive care facilities as well as appropriate pathology and radiology backup services.

The Surgery Itself

General Considerations

An experienced scrub team is essential. Forget the nursing philosophy of "rotating teams", you need to work with your best and most familiar scrub staff nurse or sister who knows how you work. This is vital. It leads to operative harmony, less time taken and, if you believe in Newtonian mathematics and the concept of rate of change, much less time waiting for things rather than getting on with the job!

Operative Position

A great deal of confusion exists amongst surgical trainees concerning the correct positioning of patients for transabdominal pelvic surgery and it is not uncommon for patients to be placed in the lithotomy position. This position provides access to the perineal organs such as the anal canal and vagina, but is incorrect for major pelvic excisions. The correct position is the Lloyd-Davies position with a wedge beneath the buttocks (Fig. 3.4). Failure to use a wedge, which is another common mistake, only serves to make access more difficult.

Preliminary Laparotomy and Assessment

A long midline incision from xiphisternum to symphysis pubis provides the best access to the abdominal and pelvic viscera. It also has the advantage of preserving the rectus abdominis muscle and its vessels in case the surgeon needs to utilise this muscle for myocutaneous reconstruction.

The mobility and extent of local invasion should be accurately assessed for these are factors that deem whether or not the primary tumour is curable. Usually tumour fixation and infiltration into the pelvic side walls is obvious. However, in the male with a narrow pelvis, there may be "pseudofixation". This refers to a bulky primary lesion that has not infiltrated surrounding tissues but which limited in its mobility by the confines of the bony pelvis. Some clue to this phenomenon can be revealed by reviewing preoperative imaging during the course of the operation.

The assessment of transcoelomic spread is particularly important when taken in conjunction with the type of tumour, its anticipated biological behaviour and potential response to adjuvant chemoradiotherapy. For example, there is little value in resecting the rectum, bladder and perineum in a patient with primary or

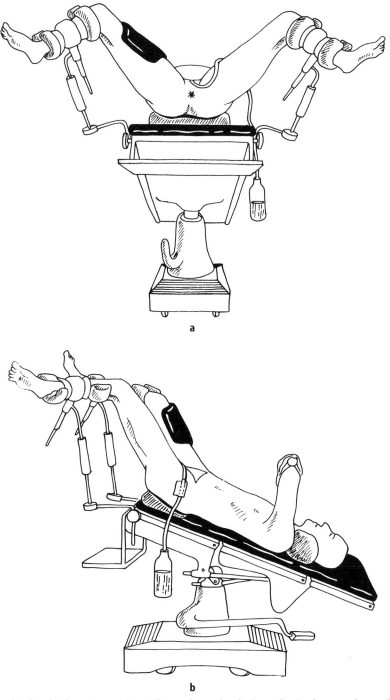

a

b

Fig. 3.4a,b. The Lloyd-Davies position with a wedge under the buttocks. (Redrawn and reproduced with permission, from Surgery of the Anus, Rectum and Colon, by Michael R.B. Keighley and Norman S. Williams, WB Saunders Co., March 1994, ISBN 0702012785)

recurrent carcinoma of the rectum in the presence of extensive peritoneal spread of tumour because at this stage rectal cancers are unlikely to respond to any kind of adjuvant treatment. To undertake extensive resection under these circumstances simply serves to reduce the quality of the patients remaining life. By contrast, the situation is quite the reverse in ovarian cancer.[2,3,4,15,28-31] Aggressive resection of the primary tumour and related structures together with peritoneal deposits can reduce the bulk of a potentially chemosensitive tumour to a level where adjuvant treatment can produce a significant and good quality prolongation of life.

Techniques of Resection

Careful assessment by laparotomy and operability should allow the surgeons to decide whether the operation will be palliative or potentially curative. In either event the aim is to achieve total "en bloc" excision of the tumour and involved organs. It is impossible to cover every aspect of resection, but some general guidelines can be provided and these are best considered anatomically moving from a cephalad to a caudal direction. Moreover, in practice it does not matter whether the dissection proceeds from anterior to posterior or vice versa. However, it should be remembered that mobilisation of the bladder allows better access to the posterior pelvis.

The Pelvic Brim

This can be one of the most difficult areas in this type of surgery because of the proximity of the common and external iliac vessels. Localised involvement of the iliac artery should not deter excision of the vessel and vascular reconstruction if this allows potential clearance of tumour. Venous involvement should be treated by ligation of the iliac vein proximally and distally. Primary venous reconstruction is seldom necessary and may be unduly dangerous. Arterial injury can be managed by repair whilst venous injury carries grave consequences. One or both ureters may require division at this level and the internal iliac vessels can be sacrificed with impunity.

If the ureters are involved in a rectal cancer then it is usually necessary to remove the bladder (and prostate in a man) even if the cancer is not obviously invading the bladder base itself. Preservation of part of the bladder with subsequent bladder augmentation cystoplasty and ureteric reimplantation is sometimes possible. Alternatively even a radical prostatectomy and "en bloc" proctosigmoidectomy is possible.[32] However, preoperative and even peroperative staging are not accurate to a tolerance of millimetres and such a conservative approach to ablation is bound to be accompanied by relatively higher cancer recerrence rates.[5]

Lower Down in the Pelvis

Surgical strategy now depends on the extent of exenteration planned: i.e. posterior, anterior or total, and a decision should have also been reached concerning the necessity for sacrifice of the levator plate and perineum. Anteriorly, the inferior vesical pedicle should be exposed and divided last because control may be lost here and it is necessary to remove the surgical specimen in order to control the bleeding. The lateral dissection seldom presents any major problems.

The posterior dissection depends to a large extent on the situation of the tumour. With retrorectal tumours, recurrent rectal carcinoma and primary rectal cancers that have invaded posteriorly, dissection proceeds along a plane clear of the tumour mass, which is usually posterior to the plane of resection of more localised rectal cancers, i.e. immediately behind the mesorectum in front of the hypogastric nerves. As a result of this, bleeding from presacral veins can be problematical. Whilst it may be necessary to deal with this by packing, the insertion of sterile drawing pins into the presacral foramina is a useful manoeuvre and usually successful in quelling haemorrhage. The division of Waldeyer's fascia is a vital manoeuvre for delivering the contents of the posterior pelvis.

Some tumours may invade the lower sacrum and this can be resected in continuity with posterior or total pelvic exenteration.[16,33] If the bladder is to remain, then partial sacral excision with preservation of S3 nerve roots is all that is feasable. However, if the exenteration involves removal of the bladder as well, subtotal sacrectomy may be performed. Under these circumstances, the abdominal parts of the operation should be completed, the patient turned and the posterior excision performed from the back.

The Perineum

On the basis of preoperative staging and assessment of the extent of tumour spread at operation, a decision regarding the extent of perineal excision should have been reached. In practice this may range from removal of the anal canal to wide perineal excision including part or all of the vulva and vagina in the female or scrotum and penile base in the male.

Peritoneal Deposits and other Intra-abdominal Organs

The necessity for extended resection in the abdomen usually occurs with ovarian tumours where multiple "mass" lesions as opposed to miliary type of spread may be present throughout the abdomen and may involve just about any viscera.[3] Providing that the primary tumour is chemosensitive, then resection of these deposits can justly be performed as part of a "cytoreductive debulking" procedure. There are no hard and fast rules and the extent of resection necessary will be governed by the particular situation encountered. However, with ovarian tumours, the surgeon should pay special attention to the undersurface of the diaphragm because deposits here are common and easily excised.

Reconstruction

General Principles

The avoidance of a stoma is a secondary consideration to complete tumour clearance and if oncologically indicated, urinary and faecal stomas should be constructed carefully at sites which have been marked preoperatively. More recently, there has been a trend away from "double diversion" after radical pelvic surgery in favour of reconstruction of one or both systems.[34–37] There is evidence of significantly improved quality of life when an aggressive reconstructive approach is taken.[27] Other issues which require consideration are the creation of a neovagina in the female and reconstruction of the pelvic floor and perineum.

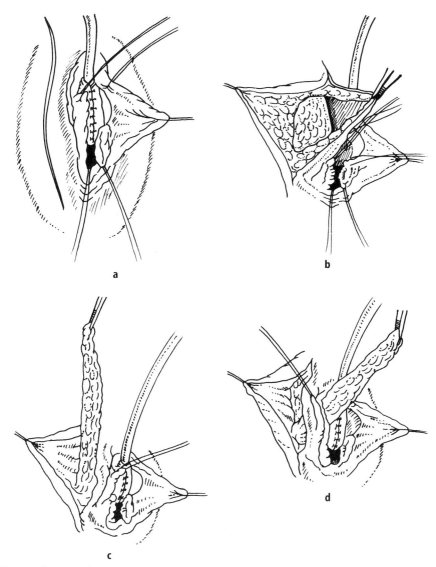

Fig. 3.5a–d. Series of drawings to show the mobilisation of a labial fat pad. **a** Longitudinal incision is made on the medial aspect of the labium majorus. **b** The yellow pad of fat is dissected off the underlying pubis and freed from it anterior attachment to form a finger of tissue **c, d** Based on the posterior vessels, this is then rotated into the vaginal defect.

Any visceral reconstruction in the pelvis ought to be protected by mobilisation of the greater omentum away from the greater curvature of the stomach based on the left gastroepiploic artery. This can then be wrapped around or laid across any anastomoses and particularly where those of the faecal and urinary systems lie in close proximity. If greater omentum is not available in the female (for instance where it has had to be sacrificed to achieve cancer clearance in extensive ovarian disease) a useful manoeuvre to obtain extra healthy fatty tissue is the Martius fat graft. The skin of the labia majora is incised to reveal a large fatty pedicle which, based on the pudendal vessels, can be rotated into the pelvis and used to interpose between suture lines (Fig. 3.5a–d).

Colorectal Reconstruction

From the practical point of view, colorectal anastomoses should precede vaginal or urinary reconstruction because access posterior to either of these is usually difficult or impossible. Continuity can be achieved by a standard colorectal anastomosis if the distal rectum is left in situ. However, if the rectum is transected at the anorectal junction, then coloanal anastomosis is necessary using a stapled or handsewn peranal technique.[38,39] Traditionally, coloanal anastomoses have been fashioned in an end-to-end manner, but the use of coloanal J pouch anastomosis[40,41] is gaining in popularity. There is increasing evidence to suggest that coloanal pouch anastomosis is associated with a lower rate of anastomotic failure than straight anastomosis and that postoperative function is improved.[40] In an attempt to improve postoperative function further, von Flue et al.[42] have described reversed ileocaecal interposition between the descending colon and the top of the anal canal.

All colorectal or coloanal anastomoses are vulnerable to overt failure and it is good practice to wrap them with greater omentum if this structure has been preserved. Moreover, this manoeuvre will reduce the likelihood of fistulation between colorectal or coloanal and urinary or neo-vaginal anastomoses. Further consideration should be given to the need for temporary faecal diversion in the form of loop ileostomy or colostomy.

Urinary Tract Reconstruction

The basic decision that needs to be made is to choose between in situ "orthotopic" reconstruction or urinary diversion. The latter may be incontinent with an ileal conduit or continent with a catheterisable stoma. The choice between reconstruction or diversion depends on what structures and tissues are still available following ablative resection, on the patient's condition having reached that point in the surgery and, not least, on the wishes of the patient, which will have been evaluated preoperatively. The long-term complications of urinary reconstruction must be borne in mind when making these decisions. In addition, if the operation has been only palliative locally, and this may require confirmation by frozen section of nodes or pelvic side wall at the time, then complex reconstruction is unwise. Local tumour recurrence or the need for early adjuvant radiotherapy may impair healing of anastomoses and adversely affect the function of the reconstructed organ. Moreover, if a complicated colorectal reconstruction has been performed, or if the patient's peroperative condition is poor, then it may be better to create a temporary ileal conduit with a view to converting this to an orthotopic reconstruction at a later date.

There are several situations which may be encountered urologically and it is convenient to consider them separately.

If the Urethra is Normal

If the urethra and external sphincter mechanism is still in place and is expected to function normally, a substitution cystoplasty or "orthotopic reconstruction" provides excellent results. The aim is to provide a good capacity, low-pressure reservoir for urine storage, to protect the upper urinary tracts if possible by preventing reflux and to provide urinary continence during bladder-filling but normal voiding through the urethra and complete emptying of the neobladder.

The ingenuity of surgeons in designing new and varied methods of "sewing a bag" and a "couple of valves" from a tube of bowel is quite remarkable. Even more astounding is that many surgeons always appear to perform diversions or reconstructions in the same way. This is not our experience. The ease with which one particular loop of bowel can be reconfigured and laid into the pelvis varies from one patient to another and it is vital for the surgeon to have a number of surgical tricks up his or her sleeve. This does not make for a "clean" operative series, but does mean that solutions are tailored more to the patient's particular problems. Textbook training is no substitute for sound technique, which will only be acquired by apprenticeship, flexibility in decision making and above all experience.

The reservoir can made be in countless ways by using a "pouch" of intestine which may be constructed from 40+ cm of ileum, an ileocaecal pouch or a colonic pouch. There has been much debate about whether the pouch should be detubularised to create U, N or W shaped configurations. The advantage, theoretically, is that increasing numbers of folds will more nearly approximate a sphere, thus resulting in the best capacity for a given surface area. In addition the effect of contractions of circular muscle of the bowel wall is diminished, which produces better compliance. Unfortunately, in practice the theoretical physical advantages outlined above are not always achieved. By contrast, tubular segments of right colon can be made into a neobladder faster and with less blood loss than a detubularisation (Fig. 3.6), which is a major advantage after bloody ablative surgery. They also provide better pouch emptying, although with higher rates of night-time incontinence caused by higher resting pressures.[43] Absorbable stapling devices will help to shorten operating times for making a detubularised pouch.

Supratrigonal substitution or augmentation cystoplasty with a small bowel segment may be justified if it has been possible to preserve the bladder trigone and both ureters. Paradoxically, however, the rates of reflux after supratrigonal cystoplasty are higher and this is presumably because of distortion of the intravesical segment of the ureter during suturing of the cystoplasty, whilst with a total substitution the ureters are consciously reimplanted.

Continence of the outlet of the neobladder is best provided by the native urethral sphincter.[44] If the urethral sphincter is compromised, a detubularised substitution cystoplasty is essential to allow low enough resting pressures and a greater capacity. In women it may be necessary to augment sphincter closure or bladder

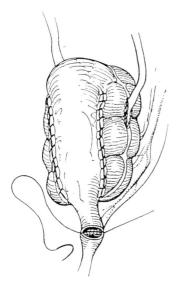

Fig. 3.6. Drawing to show the principle of an orthotopic bladder reconstruction using an ileocaecal detubularised pouch. The ureters are implanted through a taenia each whilst the most proximal segment of ileum has been left unopened and is rotated to be anastomosed to the proximal urethra. (Reproduced with permission, from Light and Scardino (1986) Urol Clin North Am 13:261–270.)

neck support by concomitant placement of a simple periurethral sling or by approximation of the anterior vaginal wall tissues to the obturator fascia or pectineal ligament as for a conventional retropubic anti-incontinence procedure. This is particularly so if there was preoperative urogenital prolapse or if it is felt that the ablative surgery has compromised normal sphincter function. An artificial sphincter cuff can be inserted and left deactivated until the patient has recovered from surgery when the remaining working parts of the device can be inserted.[43] Occasionally this will be unnecessary because the cuff itself provides enough outlet resistance to prevent leakage. However, this would rarely be appropriate in the context of radical ablative cancer surgery.

If the Urethra has been Removed

Whilst it is possible to reconstruct the urethra in a female with a labial skin tube this would rarely be contemplated if rectal reconstruction was also taking place. These patients require a urinary diversion whether it be continent or incontinent.

Urinary Diversion. Bricker[45] first described in 1950 the creation of the ileal conduit to create an incontinent abdominal stoma for urinary diversion and the technique has evolved little since that time. The operation is technically simple compared with other reconstructive options and offers reliability and a low likelihood of reoperation. However, there are significant complications including parastomal hernia, stomal prolapse and fistula, infection and stone formation. Apparent upper tract deterioration over several years occurs and may be related to the fact that the bowel segment used is tubular, develops high segmental pressures during peristalsis and is usually refluxing . Ileal conduits should be short, and are best laid through the mesentery of the small bowel, which facilitates both a tension free stoma and the shortest length possible. The ureteroileal anastomosis is best placed above the level of the pelvic brim so that postoperative radiotherapy is less likely to impair healing. If a significant length of ureter has been lost on one side, then either a transuretero-ureterostomy can be made. Alternatively a longer piece of ileum may be used that will lie across the retroperitoneum and accept ureteric implantation at separate sites. Continent urinary diversion follows the same principles as neobladder formation but simply places the outlet on the abdominal wall rather than using the urethra. A catheterisable stoma can be placed virtually anywhere on the abdominal wall to facilitate catheterisation. Virtually any intra-abdominal tube can be used to create a catheterisable stoma.[46] The commonest used are the appendix , tapered small bowel and ureter, in association with a transuretero-ureterostomy. The appendix, provided it can be catheterised, is the most reliable of these and can almost always be made to lie in a position that will both implant generously into the neobladder and yet reach the skin.[47,48] Tapered tubes work well but are more likely to lead to difficulties with catheterisation that may need further surgery to rectify. The continence mechanism may employ either a flap valve mechanism or a hydraulic principle in which the filling pressure of the bladder itself compressed the catheterised stoma. Failure of the continence mechanism is one of the commonest early complications of these operations. The most widely used operations have been the appendiceal "Mitroffanoff" procedure (Fig. 3.7) , the Kock pouch[35] and the Indiana pouch.[49]

New techniques of ureteric implantation, antibiotics, better suture materials and development of pouches with low pressure urodynamics have led to a resurgence of interest in rectal bladders,[50] particularly in parts of the world where stoma bags are either unavailable or culturally unacceptable. The sigmoid rectal pouch uses a side-to-side linking of the sigmoid posteriorly, a nipple or submucosal tunnel implantation of the ureters and an anterior formation of a rectosigmoid pouch.[51] Whilst this obviously requires a good sphincter beforehand, authors have presented high continence rates.

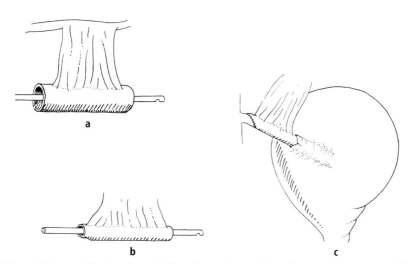

Fig 3.7a–c. Diagram indicating the principles of a continent urinary diversion. **a** A segment of ileum has been mobilised on its vascular pedicle. **b** It has been tapered to form a narrow catheterisable tube. **c** It is then implanted though a submucosal tunnel into the pouch. (Reproduced with permission, from Woodhouse and Macneilly (1994), Blackwell Science Ltd., Br J Urol 74:447–453.)

Wet colostomy, where the ureters are simply implanted into an end-colostomy is a poor substitute for double stomas as it is very difficult to look after without leakage and excoriation and also because of the very high rates of urinary infection.[52] A double-barrelled wet colostomy has been described that may circumvent some of these problems.[53,54]

When making a decision about the type of reconstruction to be employed there are a number of complications of incorporating bowel into the urinary tract which should be considered in the context of the underlying diagnosis and the likelihood of cure. In general the longer bowel mucosa spends in contact with stored urine the greater these problems tend to be. The use of an ileal segment causes intestinal hurry due to disruption of bile acid metabolism, metabolic acidosis, altered calcium metabolism and vitamin B_{12} deficiency. High-pressure pouches pose a threat to upper renal tract function. The increased urinary excretion of calcium phosphate and magnesium together with mucus and infection leads to stone formation in about 40% of patients. Mucus, from the ileal mucosa, is often a nuisance and may cause urethral and catheter blockage. Finally, there is a theoretical risk of malignancy in the reconstructed bladder though this is a minor consideration in patients undergoing this type of surgery.

The debate about which reconstruction is best also revolves around reported complication rates. These are, of course, highly dependent on surgical technique so it is unwise to extrapolate the experience of others to one's own practice. Many individual series have been presented and usually reflect the bias of the authors. A number of "comparisons" of technique can be found in the literature but none of these are randomised trials, so the differences reflect as much about patient selection as they do about the particular techniques employed. There seems little doubt that complication rates from continent diversions, whilst numerically not much different to the ileal conduit or orthotopic reconstruction, are more complex and difficult to resolve. The Kock pouch[35] seems to be fraught with trouble compared with the appendiceal diversion or the Indiana pouch. Orthotopic reconstruction, provided the patient is independent enough to use his or her own urethra for voiding, provides the best functional outcome, with lower complication rates than continent diversion but higher than for ileal conduit.

Vaginal Reconstruction

Vaginal reconstruction can be performed at the time of the initial operation or as a delayed procedure.[5] Visceral substitution with small or large bowel can be employed to create a mucus-producing tube. Colon works much better than small bowel[55] because it has an intrinsic muscular rigidity. If the whole right colon has been mobiliised along with terminal ileum, an ileocolonic pouch can be used for the bladder reconstruction whilst the distal 15 cm or so of the colonic segment can be mobilised on a vascular pedicle and rotated in between the rectum and neobladder. Alternatively, a variety of myocutaneous flaps such as rectus abdominis,[56,57] gluteus maximus, gracilis and bulbocavernosus can be fashioned into tubular structures in order to create a neo-vagina.[5,58]

Pelvic Floor and Perineum

The surgeon should, on the basis of preoperative staging, have determined how much of the pelvic floor and soft issues of the perineum need to be sacrificed. It is unlikely that if reconstruction of either the colorectum or urinary tract is to be undertaken that reconstitution of the pelvic floor needs to be considered. However, when the surgeon is dealing with recurrent rectal cancer, vaginal cancer, vulval cancer, extensive squamous cancers anywhere in the perineum and uncommon soft tissue sarcomas, pelvic floor and perineal reconstruction become an integral consideration in the overall "game plan" for surgery. It should be understood that pelvic floor reconstruction is undertaken to prevent herniation of viscera through the pelvic diaphragm whilst perineal closure is performed to provide soft tissue cover in order that healing may occur as rapidly as possible.

Pelvic Floor Reconstruction

After excision of all or some of the pelvic viscera, it is seldom possible to close the pelvic peritoneum. The greater omentum can be used to close the defect being loosely sutured to the pelvic sidewalls to prevent dislocation in the immediate postoperative period. However if there has been reconstruction of more than one viscera the omentum has a much more important role in protecting anastomoses and it should be preserved for this purpose. In this situation, or if omentum is not available, absorbable or non-absorbable meshes may be used,[59] or alternatively one of the muscle flaps (without skin) as described below. The use of Dura mater has also been reported[60] but the present authors have no personal experience of this technique.

Perineal Reconstruction

Muscle transposition with or without a skin paddle provides an ideal method of filling large perineal defects which result from surgery. If a skin island is included immediately, then the cutaneous defect may be closed at the same time. However, it is the authors' practice to use primary muscle transposition followed by delayed split skin grafting. The types of muscle flap available can be classified in several ways but the rectus abdominis muscle is the most commonly used abdominal flap and is particularly suited to reconstructing major defects in the anterior perineum and pelvic floor.[61] The muscle is mobilised using the inferior epigastric vessels as the basis for the pedicle. It should be remembered that abdominal closure may be compromised after the use of this type of muscle flap and due consideration should be given to stoma siting during preoperative planning. If two stomas are being considered then it is better to use a different flap.[62]

There are various permutations and combinations of buttock and thigh muscles which can be used and these include gluteus maximus, vastus medialis, sartorius and gracilis.[62] The authors have found that bilateral gracilis transposition provides a useful method of reconstructing perineal defects.

In keeping with a multidisciplinary approach to these problems, it is beneficial to involve a plastic surgeon as a member of the surgical team.

Outcome

Perioperative Morbidity and Mortality

Improvements in patient selection and better pre- and postoperative care have led to a reduction in perioperative mortality from 20–30% in the 1950s[9,12,63] to less than 10% in the current decade.[64–68] Nevertheless, total or partial pelvic exenteration still carries a considerable morbidity which ranges from 32 to 84%. Some of these postoperative complications are the inevitable sequelae of any major intra-abdominal procedure, but others are specifically related to complex colorectal, urinary and sometimes vascular reconstruction. The balance between the increased likelihood of specific complications and morbidity as the result of complex reconstruction and lesser procedures such as "double diversion" should be considered very carefully by the surgical team. Moreover, previous pelvic radiotherapy has been shown by several authors to increase perioperative morbidity.[1,2,9,11,24,28,38]

Survival

The very nature of these tumours means that most series that report outcome are retrospective and often based on small numbers of patients. This lack of prospective data makes the meaningful analysis of long-term survival figures difficult to establish after pelvic exenteration. Case selection is rarely explicit in such reports and one never knows how many patients were refused surgery. In one series of 1000 patients being considered for radical resectional surgery, only 20% were deemed suitable for operation.

The reported morbidity, mortality and survival in many larger series is variable (Table 3.2). What is clear from these studies is that long-term outcome will depend largely on the type and biological behaviour of the tumour, and to a lesser

Table 3.2. Perioperative morbidity, mortality and survival after pelvic exenteration for locally advanced malignancies

Author	Year	Site	n	Morbidity	Mortality	5-year survival
Kiselow[13]	1967	M	312		7.8	30–35
Symmonds[63]	1975	M	198			
Rutledge[14]	1977	G	296			33–42
Boey[24]	1982	CR	49		27	28–52
Jakowatz[64]	1985	M	104	49	2.9	27
Lindsey[65]	1985	M	68		4.4	33
Kraybill[29]	1988	M	99		14	45
Lawhead[30]	1989	G	65		9.2	23
Shingleton[15]	1989	G	143		6.3	42–63
Soper[67]	1989	M	69	38	7.2	
Hafner[16]	1992	CR	75	75	5	43
Yeung[25]	1993	CR	50	71	14	10
Lopez[18]	1994	M	232	45	10	42
Wanebo[68]	1994	CR	53		8.5	18
Hida[17]	1998	CR	50	22	6	60–80

CR, colorectal pathology; M, mixed pathologies (gynaecological, colorectal and sarcomas); G, gynaecological pathology.

extent on the radicality of the original resection and the use of adjuvant radio-therapy and chemotherapy.

References

1. Avradopoulos KA, Vezeridis MP, Wanebo RJ (1996) Pelvic exenteration for recurrent rectal cancer. Adv Surg. 29:215–33.
2. Bridges J, Oram D (1993) Management of advanced gynaecological malignancies. Br J Hosp Med 49:191–199.
3. Franchi M, Donadello N (1994) Pelvic exenteration in gynecologic oncology. Eur J Gynecol Oncol 15:469–474.
4. Rogo KO, Stendahl U (1993) Management of recurrent cervical cancer:the place of ultraradical surgery. East Afr Med J 70:380– 385.
5. Rodriguez-Bigas MA, Petrelli NJ (1996) Pelvic exenteration and its modifications. Am J Surg 171:293–301.
6. Tarraza HM, Ellerkmann RM (1998) Pelvic radical surgery. Surg Oncol Clin North Am 7:399–416.
7. Magrina JF (1993) Complications of irradiation and radical surgery for gynaecologic malignan-cies. Obstet Gynecol Surv 48:571–575.
8. Saunders N (1995) Pelvic exenteration: by whom and for whom? Lancet 345:5–6.
9. Brunschwig A (1948) Complete excision of pelvic viscera for advanced carcinoma. Cancer 1:177–183.
10. Brintnall ES, Flocks RH (1950) "En masse" pelvic viscerectomy with ureterointestinal anastomo-sis. Arch Surg. 61:851–864.
11. Bricker EM, Modlin J (1951) The role of pelvic evisceration in surgery. Surgery 30:76–94.
12. Brunschwig A (1956) Pelvic exenteration for carcinoma of the lower colon. Surgery 40:691–695.
13. Kiselow M, Butcher HR, Bricker EM (1967) Results of the radical treatment of advanced pelvic cancer: a 15-year study. Ann Surg 166:428–436.
14. Rutledge FN, Smith JP, Wharton JT et al. (1977) Pelvic exenteration: analysis of 296 patients. Am J Obstet Gynecol 129:881–892.
15. Shingleton HM, Soong SJ, Getter MS et al. (1989) Clinical and histopathological factors predicting recurrence and survival after pelvic exenteration for cancer of the cervix. Obstet Gynecol 73:1077–1034.
16. Hafner GH, Herrera L, Petrelli NJ (1991) Patterns of recurrence after pelvic exenteration for colorectal carcinoma. Arch Surg 126:1510–1513.
17. Hida J, Yasutomi M, Maruyama T et al. (1998) Results from pelvic exenteration for locally advanced colorectal cancer with lymph node metastases. Dis Colon Rectum 41:165–168.
18. Lopez MJ, Standford SB, Skibba JI (1994) Total pelvic exenteration. Arch Surg 120:390–396.
19. Marshall FF, Treiger BF (1991) Radical cystectomy (anterior exenteration) in the female patient. Urol Clin North Am 18:765–775.
20. Kevwitch MK, Walloch JL, Waters WB, Flanigan RC (1993) Prostatic cystic epithelial-stromal tumours: a report of 2 new cases. J Urol 149:860–864.
21. Hicks BA, Hensle TW, Burbige KA, Altman RP (1993) Bladder management in children with genitourinary sarcoma. J Pediatr Surg 28:1019–1022.
22. Reid CG, Morley GW, Schmidt RW et al. (1989) The role of pelvic exenteration for sarcomatous malignancies. Obstet Gynecol 74:80–84.
23. Takagi H, Morimoto T, Kato T et al. (1983) Pelvic exenteration combined with sacral resection for recurrent rectal cancer. J Surg Oncol 24:161–166.
24. Boey J, Wong J (1982) Pelvic exenteration for locally advanced colorectal carcinoma. Ann Surg 195:513–518.
25. Yeung RS, Moffat FL, Falk RE (1993) Pelvic exenteration for recurrent and extensive primary colorectal adenocarcinoma. Cancer 72:1853–1858.
26. Holmes SA, Christmas TJ, Kirby RS, Hendry WF (1992) Management of colovesical fistulae associated with pelvic malignncy. Br J Surg 79:432–434.
27. Hawighorst-Knapstein S, Shonefuss G, Hoffman SO, Knapstein PG (1997) Pelvic exenteration: effects of surgery on quality of life and body image – a prospective longitudinal study. Gynecol Oncol 66:495–500.
28. DiSaia P, Creaseman WT (1984) Invasive cervical cancer. In: DiSaia P, Creaseman WT (eds) Clinical gynaecologic oncology, 2nd edn. Mosby, St Louis, pp 61–125.

29. Kraybill WG. Lopez MJ. Bricker EM (1988) Total pelvic exenteration as a therapeutic option in advanced malignant disease of the pelvis. Surg Obstet Gynecol 166:259–263.

30. Lawhead RA Jr, Clark DG, Smith DH, Pierce VK, Lewis JL Jr (1989) Pelvic exenteration for recurrent or persistent gynecologic malignancies: a 10-year review of the Memorial Sloan-Kettering Cancer Center experience (1972–1981). Gynecol Oncol 33:279–282.

31. Robertson G, Lopes A, Beynon G, Monaghan JM (1994) Pelvic exenteration: a review of the Gateshead experience 1974–1992. Br J Obstet Gynecol 101:529–531.

32. Campbell SC, Church JM, Fazio VW, Klein EA, Pontes JE (1993) Combined radical retropubic prostatectomy and proctosigmoidectomy for en bloc removal of locally invasive carcinoma of the rectum. Surg Gynecol Obstet 176:605–608.

33. Maetani S, Onodera T, Nishikawa T et al. (1998) Significance of local recurrence of rectal cancer as a local or disseminated disease. Br J Surg 85:521–525.

34. Goluboff ET, McKiernan JM,Todd G, Nowygrod R, Smith D, Olsson CA (1994) Reconstruction of urinary and gastrointestinal tracts in total pelvic exenteration: experience at Columbia Presbyterian Medical Center. Urology 44:666–670.

35. Skinner DG, Sherrod A (1990) Total pelvic exenteration with simultaneous bowel and urinary reconstruction. J Urol 144:1438–1439.

36. Shepherd JH, Crawford RAF, Christmas TJ, Hendry WF (1997) Total pelvic reconstruction after exenteration for recurrent cervical cancer. Br J Urol 80 (Suppl 1):79–81.

37. Skinner DG, Boyd SD, Lieskovsky G, Bennett C, Hopwood B (1991) Lower urinary tract reconstruction following cystectomy: experience and results in 126 patients using the Kock ileal reservoir with bilateral ureteroileal urethrostomy. J Urol 146:756–760.

38. Berek JS, Hacker NF, Lagasse LD (1984) Rectosigmoid colectomy and reanastomosis to facilitate resection of primary and recurrent gynaecological cancer. Obstet Gynecol 64:715–720.

39. Wheeless CR (1993) Low colorectal anastomosis and reconstruction after gynaecological cancer. Cancer 71:1664–1666.

40. Parc R, Tiret E, Frileux P, Moszkowki E, Loygue J (1986) Resection and coloanal anastomosis with colonic reservoir for rectal carcinoma. Br J Surg 73:139–141.

41. Williams NS (1989) Stapling technique for pouch anal anastomosis without the need for purse string suture. Br J Surg 76:348–349.

42. von Flue M, Harder F (1994) New technique for pouch-anal reconstruction after total mesorectal excision. Dis Colon Rectum 37:1160–1162.

43. Mundy AR (1993) Urodynamic and reconstructive surgery of the lower urinary tract. Churchill Livingstone. Ediburgh.

44. Woodhouse CRJ (1995) Continent urinary diversion: outlet considerations. Curr Opin Urol 5:123–126.

45. Bricker EM (1950) Bladder substitution after pelvic evisceration. Surg Clin North Am. 30:1511–1521.

46. Sumfest JM, Burns MW, Mitchell ME (1993) The Mitrofanoff Principle in urinary reconstruction. J Urol 150:1875–1877.

47. Barker SB (1991) Continent diversion with an appendix conduit and an ileocecal bladder. J Urol 146:745–754.

48. Riedmiller H (1992) Appendix as continent urinary reservoir outlet. Scand J Urol Nephrol 142:73–75.

49. Rowland RG (1996) Present experience with the Indiana Pouch. World J Urol 14:92–98.

50. Ghoneim MA (1992) The modified rectal bladder: a bladder substitute controlled by the anal sphincter. Scand J Urol Nephrol (Suppl) 142:89–91.

51. Sundin T, Mansi MK (1993) The valved "S" shaped rectosigmoid pouch for continent urinary diversion. J Urol 150:838–842.

52. Appleby LH (1950) Proctocystectomy. The management of colostomy with ureteral transplants. Am J Surg 79:57–60.

53. Osorio Gullon A, deOca J, Lopez Costea MA et al. (1997) Double-barrelled wet colostomy: a safe and simple method after pelvic exenteration. Int J Colorectal Dis 12:37–41.

54. Takada H et al. (1995) Double-barrelled wet colostomy. A simple method of urinary diversion for patients undergoing pelvic exenteration. Dis Colon Rectum 38:1325–1326.

55. Hendren WH, Atala A (1994) Use of bowel for vaginal reconstruction. J Urol 152:752–755.

56. Benson C, Soisson AP, Carlson J, Culbertson G, Rawley-Bowland C, Richards F (1993) Neovaginal reconstruction with a rectus abdominis myocutaneous flap. Obstet Gynecol 81:871–875.

57. Smith HO, Genesen MC, Runowicz CD, Goldberg GL (1998) The rectus abdominis myocutaneous flap: modifications, complications and sexual function. Cancer 83:510–520.

58. Loree TR, Hempling RE, Eltabakh GH et al. (1997) The inferior gluteal flap in the difficult vulvar and perineal reconstruction. Gynecol Oncol 66:429–433.
59. Clarke Pearson DL, Soper JT, Creasman WT (1988) Absorbable synthetic mesh (polyglactin) for the formation of a pelvic lid after radical pelvic resection. Am J Obstet Gynecol 158:158–161.
60. Jarrell MA, Malinin TI, Averette HE et al. (1987) Human Dura materallografts in repair of pelvic floor and abdominal wall defects. Obstet Gynecol 7:280–285.
61. Brough WA, Schofield PF (1991) The value of rectus abdominis myocutaneous flap in the treatment of complex perineal fistula. Dis Colon Rectum 34:148–150.
62. Keighley MRB (1993) Pesistent perineal sinus. In: Keighley MBR, Williams NS (eds) Surgery of the anus, rectum and colon. Saunders, London, pp 260–264.
63. Symmonds RE, Pratt JH, Webb MJ (1975) Exenterative operations: experience with 198 patients. Am J Obstet Gynecol 121:907–918.
64. Jakowatz JG, Porudominski D, Riihimaki DU et al. (1985) Complications of pelvic exenteration. Arch Surg 120:1261–1265.
65. Lindsey WF, Wood DK, Briele HA (1985) Pelvic exenteration. J Surg Oncol 30:231–234.
66. Morely GW, Hopkins MP, Lindenauer SM, Roberts JA (1989) Pelvic exenteration, University of Michigan:100 patients at 5 years. Obstet Gynecol 74:934–943.
67. Soper JT, Berchuk A, Creasman WT (1989) Pelvic exenteration:factors associated with major surgical morbidity. Gynecol Oncol 35:93–98.
68. Wanebo HJ, Koness RJ, Vezeridis MP, Cohen SI, Wrobleski DE (1994) Pelvic resection of recurrent rectal cancer. Ann Surg 220:586–597.

4 The Surgical Management of Crohn's Disease of the Colon

A. Allan and P.E. Bearn

Introduction

Despite advances in medical therapy for patients with colonic Crohn's disease, the majority still require operative intervention at some stage if followed up for long enough.[1,2] The management of these patients provides a challenge for the surgeon, requiring not only clinical and operative expertise but also the more traditional skill of forming a strong doctor–patient relationship. Careful counselling and the explanation of alternative surgical strategies together with their likely outcome is essential in treating these patients, and this is greatly facilitated by the recent introduction of a multidisciplinary team approach, including stoma therapist, coloproctology specialist nurse and clinical psychologist.

The behaviour of colonic Crohn's disease is closely related to its anatomical site. Right-sided disease, which is usually associated with significant ileal involvement, causes obstructive symptoms. In a series reported from Birmingham[3] 89% of cases of right-sided colonic Crohn's disease required operation. Extensive colonic disease required resection in 79% of cases, whereas Crohn's disease of the left colon was less likely to require operation (62%). When patients with Crohn's proctitis were considered, surgery was only necessary in 32% of cases. Many cases of proctitis may remain indolent for years[4] and are associated with a clinical picture often dominated by coexisting perianal Crohn's disease.[5] Furthermore, there is some evidence to suggest that chronic complicated anorectal Crohn's disease is particularly liable to malignant change.[6]

This chapter examines the common and less common indications for surgery in patients with colonic Crohn's disease. It assesses the objectives of surgical treatment and examines some unresolved problem areas such as the optimal role of faecal diversion and avoidance of inadvertent ileoanal pouch formation in patients with colonic Crohn's disease.

Indications for Surgery in Patients with Colonic Crohn's Disease

Indications for operation in patients with colonic Crohn's disease are subdivided on the basis of their relative urgency. Emergency operations are carried out within a few hours, once the patient's condition can be optimised. Urgent operations are done on the next routine operating list and elective operations at the mutual convenience of patient and surgeon.

Emergency Surgery

Indications for emergency operation include toxic dilatation of the colon. The incidence of toxic dilatation in patients with severe acute Crohn's colitis is reported to occur in between 4 and 6.3%,[7-9] and colonic Crohn's disease may progress rapidly to toxic dilatation especially in patients with a short history as well as rectal sparing.[10] Toxic dilatation virtually never occurs now in patients who are treated as inpatients with acute Crohn's colitis, but is seen occasionally in patients who are admitted with established toxic dilatation and who have ignored their symptoms. Further indications for emergency surgery may develop in patients with or without acute dilatation of the colon. These comprise colonic perforation as well as unremitting rectal haemorrhage. In the case of a patient with profuse rectal haemorrhage the possibility of a coexisting peptic ulcer bleed should be considered as these patients may be both stressed and on large doses of steroids. Those patients requiring emergency surgery for such severe colonic disease are best treated by colectomy with terminal ileostomy and preservation of the rectal stump.

Urgent Surgery

The most common indication for urgent surgery in patients with Crohn's disease of the colon is for acute severe colitis not responding to intensive intravenous steroid therapy. Patients will require colectomy if they do not respond to such treatment within a week of intensive medical therapy.[11] The exact timing of this will depend on several factors, including the patient's acceptance that an operation is the safest option. The outcome in these patients is likely to be optimal if a surgeon works closely with the medical gastroenterologist, stoma therapist and coloproctology specialist nurse so that the patient is well informed about impending surgery and the need for a stoma as early as possible before the operation becomes necessary. Patients who are not carefully counselled preoperatively tend to be those who find it difficult to accept a stoma postoperatively.

Predicting which patients with acute colitis will require urgent surgery is to some extent possible. Recently Travis and colleagues[12] suggested that on the third day of admission to hospital 85% of patients with more than eight stools on that day or a stool frequency between three and eight together with a C-reactive protein (CRP) of more than 45 mg/l would require colectomy on that admission. Certainly surgery for acute severe Crohn's colitis is indicated in patients who undergo 6 to 8 days of intensive intravenous steroid therapy without significant improvement or in whom actual deterioration is demonstrated.[13] The optimal role of cyclosporin therapy in preventing the need for surgery in such cases remains to be defined[12,14] but provides an alternative to colectomy at least on a temporary basis in some patients.

Patients with an acute exacerbation of Crohn's colitis are likely to be indistinguishable from patients with an acute exacerbation of ulcerative colitis and the true diagnosis may only emerge on subsequent histological analysis of the resected colon or development of small bowel disease.[15] It is important to exclude infective colitis by a series of three stool cultures, including *C. difficile* and toxin as well as ova cysts and parasites, as infective colitis may coexist in patients with Crohn's colitis, especially in patients on therapy for peptic ulcers.

In patients requiring operation for severe acute colitis a total colectomy with terminal ileostomy is again the operation of choice. The rectal stump is cross-stapled and left long enough to attach by stitches to the posterior rectus sheath below the lower end of the midline laparotomy incision. This practice appears safe except where there is impending perforation of the rectal stump and greatly facilitates subsequent proctectomy. We would not advocate total colectomy with immediate ileorectal anastomosis even under cover of a defunctioning loop ileostomy in this group of very sick patients.[16] Should the anastomosis leak serious sepsis could result despite diversion and the functional end result might be severely compromised.

A further indication for urgent operation is found in patients with right-sided Crohn's disease and associated ileal disease. Surgical excision is usually indicated when there is right-sided disease associated with sepsis. A simple intraperitoneal abscess in an accessible position can often be drained percutaneously by drainage under ultrasonic control, but a deep-seated complex abscess may require open operation, resection and drainage. An abscess in a patient with Crohn's disease may form complex cavities. Computed tomography (CT), magnetic resonance imaging (MRI) or labelled leucocyte scanning may each help to delineate the location of these preoperatively, but open surgery should be carried out if percutaneous drainage is not likely to succeed. Any open operation to drain sepsis should always include a careful search for abscess ramifications and satellites of sepsis, some of which may spread for great distances outside the peritoneal cavity. Sepsis should always be minimised wherever possible using percutaneous techniques before major interventional surgery, especially if the definitive operation is going to require one or more intestinal anastomoses.

Elective Surgery

Indications for elective surgery in patients with Crohn's colitis include failed medical treatment. The point at which medical treatment is said to have failed is relative. Often the patient made weary from protracted courses of oral and intravenous medical therapy decides that he no longer wishes to pursue such treatment, with repeated hospital admissions and prolonged convalescence. He may have spoken to other patients who have already undergone surgery for similar Crohn's disease to his own and who have derived much benefit from operative treatment. These considerations may well prompt the patient to ask whether a surgical solution is best. The surgeon will be influenced also by the state of the Crohn's disease. In patients who have recently undergone intensive in-patient treatment for acute colitis the surgeon may choose to observe the disease activity and the patient's symptoms closely. If the disease does not settle – the "smouldering case" – especially if there are exacerbations of disease activity when steroid therapy is weaned, then the patient will be advised to undergo operation.

A further factor that may influence the decision to operate will be episodes of intestinal obstruction. Often in patients with right-sided colonic disease the clinical picture is overshadowed by low small bowel obstruction and this may be the principal indication for operation. Generally patients with acute intestinal obstruction due to Crohn's disease settle on conservative management in the acute situation but only to recur. It has been suggested that one episode of intestinal obstruction in a patient with Crohn's disease is a warning to operate. Two episodes are an indication for operation and three episodes are an indictment of the surgeon for not having resected the obstructing segment.

Extraintestinal Manifestations

Although extraintestinal manifestations may not be the principal indication for surgery they may form secondary indications in cases where the indication for operation on the bowel is marginal. Sometimes even relatively quiescent Crohn's colitis may be accompanied by severe colitic arthritis,[17] which affects up to 20% of patients. Usually this is a fleeting asymmetrical arthritis of the knee joints. Less frequently the hips, ankles, wrist or elbows are involved. Usually colitic arthritis, so called because it is more common in patients with colonic rather than small bowel Crohn's disease, responds well to medical treatment, particularly steroids. Persistent or recurrent monoarticular arthritis may be an indication for colectomy. Colectomy is not effective in the treatment of ankylosing spondylitis in patients with Crohn's disease of the colon. In fact, ankylosing spondylitis may become more severe.

Skin Lesions

Erythema nodosum especially of the skin over the anterior tibial surface, may occur in approximately 5% of patients with Crohn's colitis and is the most common extraintestinal manifestation in children.[18] Further skin lesions occurring in patients with Crohn's colitis include pyoderma gangrenosum, which usually occurs on the lower limbs as well as areas of trauma or needle puncture sites. For erythema nodosum either mesalazine or steroid therapy is effective, whereas early lesions of pyoderma gangrenosum may respond to cyproheptadine therapy.[19] If all other measures fail and the severity of these skin lesions justifies an invasive approach then colectomy may heal them.

Eye Lesions

Episcleritis may occur in patients with Crohn's colitis[20] and may improve following colectomy. However, it is seldom more than a cause of mild periorbital itching and is therefore not likely to be an indication for surgery. Unfortunately the more severe but less common uveitis, which presents with blurring of vision and headaches, is not improved by colectomy.[21]

Other Indications for Surgery

There is an increased incidence of nephrolithiasis in patients with colonic Crohn's disease and the pathogenesis is multifactorial. Although colectomy increases the incidence of stones in patients with colonic Crohn's disease,[22] ureteric calculus may nonetheless be an indication for ureterolithotomy on occasion. In patients with Crohn's disease, amyloid deposition is a rare but well-recognised cause of death.[23] Amyloid deposition can be found in up to 25% of patients with Crohn's disease coming to post-mortem.[24] The amyloid deposition may cause a nephrotic type syndrome and renal failure.[25] A case has been reported[26] in which renal amyloidosis in a patient with colonic Crohn's disease remitted following colectomy.

Haematological complications, such as autoimmune haemolytic anaemia may very occasionally occur in patients with Crohn's colitis. Altman, 1979, reported three cases and reviewed 13 others with documented autoimmune haemolytic anaemia.[27] He recommended that high-dose steroids should be used to treat these patients but if steroid therapy did not improve the situation then splenectomy would be required and occasionally proctocolectomy has been necessary for treatment in patients not responding either to steroids or other immunosuppressive therapy.

The hepatic complications of colonic Crohn's disease do not respond to colectomy. There may be a case for orthoptic liver transplantation in young people with sclerosing cholangitis and advanced liver disease but the precise indications remain unclear.

A further group of indications for colectomy in patients with colitis due to Crohn's disease relates to prolonged use of steroids in these patients. Prolonged or repeated courses of high-dose steroids may form an indication for colectomy of themselves because of the potential side-effects of the drugs, most commonly fluid retention and osteoporosis. Some patients are intolerant of steroids in even short courses and may develop nightmares and even steroid-induced psychosis. Surgery may also be indicated because a particular patient has a relative contraindication to steroid therapy, for example, a peptic ulcer. In theory this could be overcome by the use of a steroid preparation together with a proton pump antagonist. But in practice this is seldom satisfactory.

In previous times, growth retardation in children was regarded as an indication for resectional surgery but it is now clearly understood that the cause of growth retardation is nutritional deficiency. These deficiencies occur because of poor appetite and abdominal pain which combine to reduce nutritional intake. Children with growth delay take only half the caloric requirement calculated for their height and age. When intake is supplemented to 90% of the needs for the child the rate of growth will increase from 1.8 cm annually to 6.2 cm annually after therapy.[28] Most children can be treated by enteral or possibly parenteral nutrition. Surgery is therefore occasionally indicated but only where the child is at such a state of development that time does not remain for growth before epiphysial closure.

Perianal Crohn's Disease

Perianal Crohn's disease may be a primary indication for surgery in patients with colonic Crohn's disease or else a secondary indication related to severe rectal disease that may form the main indication for operation. Generally our policy towards perianal Crohn's disease is conservative.[5] Loculating pus should be drained and anal stenosis gently dilated. Anal fistula can successfully be treated by loose Seton drainage.[29] Sometimes a loop ileostomy can be used with great benefit to treat severe perianal Crohn's disease.[30] This therapeutic conservatism is based on the observation that the natural history of perianal Crohn's disease is often indolent.[4] Sadly perianal disease may be associated with severe Crohn's proctitis, rectal stricturing and fibrosis, which may form an indication for proctectomy.[31]

The Timing of Operation and Preparation of the Patient

The optimal timing of operation is important if the best surgical results are to follow surgical intervention for colorectal Crohn's disease. In the emergency or urgent case this is a question of resuscitating and counselling the patient over a few hours or days. However, the patient who has failed to respond to intensive medical treatment over a number of months or even years may present formidable problems that must be corrected prior to major surgery. These are either nutritional, septic or psychological. Furthermore, adjuvant immunosuppression may increase the risk of complications following surgery but does not reduce the risk of recurrence. Because of this our practice is to wean these drugs slowly before operation if at all possible, although not all surgeons would agree that this is necessary.[32]

Preoperative nutritional support may be helpful in severely malnourished patients who require major colonic resection for Crohn's disease. Enteral feeding is much safer and cheaper than total parenteral nutrition and should be used initially provided it is tolerated. If not tolerated orally then nasoenteric feeding at night may be more acceptable to the patient. In malnourished patients who cannot tolerate enteral nutrition, total parenteral nutrition may be helpful in improving nutrition and preventing further nutritional depletion prior to major surgery. Malnutrition has not been shown to increase surgical morbidity except in patients requiring re-operation for postoperative enterocutaneous fistula.[33] Nutritional therapy will not reverse protein energy malnutrition if there is any severe ongoing sepsis.[34] Several studies in patients with inflammatory bowel disease suggest that up to 2 weeks of preoperative total parenteral nutrition may be useful in reversing some of the immunological abnormalities associated with malnutrition and may decrease postoperative morbidity and mortality.[35,36] However, there is no compelling evidence that more prolonged preoperative total parenteral nutrition has a beneficial effect on these patients.[37,38]

The Objectives of Surgical Treatment

The principle objectives in the surgical treatment of colonic Crohn's disease are threefold. First to relieve the patient's symptoms, second to provide the best functional results with avoidance of a permanent stoma and third to achieve these goals with a minimal recurrence rate. To some extent these factors work in opposition one to another; for example, increased length of colonic resection may correlate with increased postoperative diarrhoea, and compromise is often necessary. The relative importance of these factors may also vary greatly between patients.

The Relief of Symptoms

The surgeon needs a clear understanding of the symptoms with which the patient presents. This requires very careful history taking and is expensive in time but is essential data if the best results are to be obtained following surgery. Obstructive symptoms such as intermittent colicky abdominal pain with abdominal bloating and vomiting respond well to surgical resection of stenotic bowel, though this is not invariable. If there is doubt concerning the contribution of intestinal obstruction to the cause of symptoms, then it can be helpful to admit the patient for a trial of a "high-fibre provocation diet". This often precipitates symptoms when luminal obstruction is the underlying cause of a symptom complex that is difficult to interpret. Obstructive symptoms are the presenting complaint in the majority of the patients with colonic Crohn's disease of the right colon.[39]

Symptoms of intermittent obstruction may result from multiple fibrotic strictures due to Crohn's disease in the transverse and descending colon that will require resection. In contrast uncontrolled active Crohn's disease of the left colon may result in lethargy, weight loss or anaemia and rectosigmoid Crohn's disease may present with pericolic abscess, persistent left iliac fossa pain, together with diarrhoea and rectal bleeding. Those patients who present with symptoms of intra-abdominal abscess can often have these ameliorated by percutaneous drainage of the septic collection prior to major laparotomy.

Rectal Crohn's disease may vary in severity from mild proctitis giving rise to mild diarrhoea and bleeding to a completely destroyed, incompliant and fibrotic rectum with perianal Crohn's disease requiring urgent proctectomy to control rectal pain and debilitating faecal incontinence.

To Provide the Optimal Functional Result and Avoid Permanent Stoma Formation

In addition to relieving the patients' symptoms it is most important to provide the best functional result possible with avoidance of a permanent stoma. In contrast, creation of a temporary stoma can be a useful strategic manoeuvre in some patients. Colonic Crohn's disease very often goes into remission following faecal diversion.[40,41] In one series 75% of patients with Crohn's disease of the colon went into remission following defunctioning[41] often with a rapid general improvement in the condition of the patient. Diversion of the faecal stream is most easily be provided by a loop ileostomy,[42] which is simpler to construct and to close than a split ileostomy.[43] In addition, many cases of perianal Crohn's disease improved dramatically with defunctioning and this may make a subsequent proctectomy unnecessary. If a proctectomy does become necessary then the improvement in perianal inflammation and diminution in perineal sepsis brought about by preliminary diversion will greatly facilitate this operation.[41] The incidence of relapse of colonic Crohn's disease following restoration of continuity ranges from 28 to 60%[41,44] and appears to be greater than the relapse rate while diversion is maintained.[41]

The technique of loop ileostomy can also be used in patients with severe colonic Crohn's disease who are nutritionally severely depleted or are septic prior to a major resection. Defunctioning can be useful to delay or minimise the length of colonic resection necessary, which is an attractive option in children who tolerate the procedure well.

A few patients present with discrete short lengths of colonic Crohn's disease in an otherwise macroscopically normal colon and the functional results following segmental colonic resection in these patients is generally very satisfactory.[45] It should be remembered that an inappropriate segmental resection in the colon with more widespread disease may leave significant macroscopic disease in situ and this will give a poor functional result. For this reason segmental resection should be reserved for well-defined short skip lesions.

For most patients with colonic Crohn's disease in whom the rectal mucosa appears normal or only minimally inflamed, a total colectomy with ileorectal anastomosis should be the operation of choice. Minor degrees of rectal mucosa inflammation are not closely related to functional outcome after total colectomy and ileorectal anastomosis[46] and the important issue is to ensure that the rectum is not so inflamed that an anastomosis is hazardous. How such total colectomy with ileorectal anastomosis will function is of great importance and is related to several factors including anal sphincter competence. Decreased rectal compliance and sensation will also impair rectal function and this in turn depends upon the degree of inflammation in the rectal wall. In the immediate preoperative period patients should be able to tolerate a 150-ml distention of their rectal ampulla and should have near normal anal sphincter pressures.[47] Minor degrees of perianal Crohn's disease are not a contraindication to total colectomy and ileorectal anastomosis,[46] but patients with severe perianal Crohn's disease and active sepsis should be managed initially by a combination of local surgery to drain sepsis and topical metronidazole in the hope that the local disease can be improved. Not surprisingly, the best functional results following total colectomy and ileorectal anastomosis are to be found in young patients with rectal sparing.[48]

Following total colectomy and ileorectal anastomosis most patients will have less than six bowel actions daily whilst urgency of defecation and troublesome diarrhoea is unusual.[49,50] In a series from Leeds, 63 patients with colonic Crohn's disease were treated by total colectomy and ileorectal anastomosis.[51] Of these patients 50% had less than four actions in 24 hours and over 80% had no social restrictions; 70% felt that they needed to continue maintenance with antidiarrhoeal therapy.

When considering functional results following surgery for colonic Crohn's disease there are some patients with severe rectal disease and fibrosis in whom a panproctocolectomy would be unavoidable. It is essential to construct as optimal an ileostomy as possible in these patients because a bad ileostomy is a permanent burden on them. Good preoperative assessment by an experienced stoma therapist together with meticulous operative technique should ensure a good ileostomy. At proctocolectomy the rectal dissection can be performed as close rectal dissection or a standard mesorectal excision. It is especially important in young men to avoid damage to the pelvic sympathetic nerves in the posterior plane and the parasympathetic nerves anteriorly and laterally. In patients undergoing proctectomy for Crohn's proctitis there are often problems with perineal wound healing. The anal canal can usually be removed by an intersphincteric dissection. This will decrease the chances of delayed perineal healing. Risk factors for poor healing include severe rectal disease, active perineal disease and rectocutaneous fistulae.[52] As noted previously, in patients with a very high risk of poor perineal healing a preliminary defunctioning ileostomy may reduce the chances of complications. Otherwise in less severe cases it may be best to carry out the proctectomy but to leave the perineal skin open.

Minimal Recurrence Rates

Intensive investigation has been carried out recently in an attempt to understand the patterns and mechanisms of the recurrence of Crohn's disease following surgical resection.[53-62] There may be a marginally lower recurrence rate for colonic compared with small bowel disease, but generally no significant difference in recurrence rate has been observed when disease site is considered.[63] One study alone suggests a higher recurrence rate for colonic Crohn's disease.[64]

A new approach to study recurrence of Crohn's disease is provided by careful endoscopic studies.[65] The neoterminal ileum after ileocaecal resection is accessible to colonoscopy and a 72% recrudescence rate is reported in the neoterminal ileum 1 year following ileocaecal resection.[66-68] There appears to be no significant increase in endoscopic recurrence thereafter, suggesting that for neoterminal ileum at least, recurrence is present by 1 year or not at all. Such ileal endoscopic recurrences are highly predictive of both symptomatic and surgical recurrence rates.[66] These findings are very important when considering colonic resection with ileocolonic anastomosis. The result of which may be greatly compromised by neoterminal ileal recurrence immediately above the remaining colon.

Recently there has been great interest in the possibility that therapeutic agents may decrease the rate of recurrence of Crohn's disease following resection. A dose of 2.4–3 g/day of 5-aminosalicyclic acid (5-ASA) is known to reduce the recurrence rate of Crohn's disease following resection as assessed endoscopically up to 3 years following resection. It may be important to start the 5-ASA treatment within 2 weeks of resection to achieve the maximal reduction in recurrence rates.[60,70,71]

There is data to suggest that recurrence of ileocaecal Crohn's disease is greater in smokers when compared with non-smokers. So there is every reason for patients recovering from resections for Crohn's disease to stop smoking.[72] One study suggests that following initial resection the occurrence of postoperative complications, a reflection of immune suppression could also be a risk factor for postoperative recurrence.[61] Unfortunately other studies do not show similar findings and the result, although interesting is open to some controversy.

Re-operation rates correlate closely with both endoscopic and symptomatic recurrence.[66] Re-operation for colonic Crohn's disease depends markedly on the type of operation carried out. Patients with severe disseminated colorectal disease including rectal stricturing and fibrosis will require a panproctocolectomy. The re-operation rate for patients undergoing proctocolectomy 10 years after the initial procedure lies in the region of between 9 and 23%.[73,74] It is interesting that ileal recurrence is more common after ileorectal anastomosis than after proctocolectomy although the significance of this observation is not understood.[74]

When the rectal ampulla is spared of disease then it is possible to carry out a total colectomy with ileorectal anastomosis. Approximately 20–30% of patients with large bowel Crohn's disease are suitable for total colectomy with ileorectal anastomosis.[51,73] However, if followed up for long enough, approximately 50% of patients will eventually require rectal excision.[46,51] Accumulative re-operation rate at 10 years is 48%, which is greater than that for proctocolectomy.[46]

Some patients with colonic Crohn's disease have a short segment of colonic disease that may be resected and followed by colo-colonic anastomosis. Following such conservative operations re-operation for recurrent disease at 10 years can reach 66%.[45] This recurrence rate therefore limits the usefulness of segmental resection in the colon except in a very few highly selected cases with short lengths of colonic disease.

From these well-established studies it is clear that re-operation rates for colonic Crohn's disease are closely related to the magnitude of the resectional procedure carried out. When precise details of operative technique are considered there is general consensus that microscopic changes of Crohn's disease at resection margins do not influence either recurrence rates or re-operation rates.[53,75] Anastomotic technique appears not to influence either endoscopically detected or symptomatic recurrence rates. One prospective randomised study showed no difference in these recurrence rates between patients having ileocolonic anastomosis made end-to-end and those having ileocolonic anastomosis made side-to-side.[76] A retrospective study suggests there is also no difference in recurrence rates between patients with ileocaecal disease undergoing either side-to-side or end-to-side anastomosis.[77]

In order to achieve the best results following surgery for colonic Crohn's disease it is essential to have a good understanding preoperatively of the extent of the disease. In the elective situation this can best be done using colonoscopy with multiple colonic biopsies. A small bowel barium study may also be necessary. If an ileorectal anastomosis is considered then anorectal physiological studies will be useful. The patient's nutrition can be optimised and steroid therapy minimised prior to operation. The precise operative procedure is chosen at laparotomy and coexisting stenotic small bowel disease excluded by a suitable balloon pull-through technique. Following operation patients can be treated with 5-ASA within 2 weeks of operation and those who smoke cigarettes are urged to stop smoking in the hope of minimising recurrence rates.

Special Considerations

The Feasibility of Laparoscopic Resections for Crohn's Disease of the Colon

Since the introduction of laparoscopic cholecystectomy, surgeons have widened the application of laparoscopic techniques throughout the gastrointestinal tract. Not surprisingly resection of ileocaecal Crohn's disease has now been carried out laparoscopically in some centres and a few resections for colonic Crohn's disease have also been performed. Ludwig and colleagues[78] from the Cleveland Clinic have recently reviewed their early experience with laparoscopic techniques in the surgical treatment of Crohn's disease. These patients appear highly selected before operation. Over 2 years, 31 patients were treated laparoscopically for Crohn's disease. The majority for either ileocaecal resection or else formation of a loop stoma. For ileocaecal resection the bowel is mobilised using the laparoscope before exteriorisation and anastomosis through a small 5-cm skin incision near the umbilicus. In the Cleveland Clinic series, 10 patients had undergone previous abdominal surgery. Despite this it was possible to complete 10 of 14 ileocaecal resections laparoscopically as well as one total colectomy with ileorectal anastomosis and two segmental colonic resections. Ten of 11 loop ileostomies were also completed laparoscopically. Conversions to open surgery were brought about by dense adhesions from previous surgery, severe inflammation with mesenteric thickening and in one case each a pre-existing contained perforation or excessive small bowel dilatation. All patients undergoing resectional procedures were allowed home within 1 week and morbidity was low.

It seems from this series that it is feasible to carry out intestinal resection for Crohn's disease including both segmental or total colectomy with ileorectal anastomosis. The patients need careful selection and contraindications at present include intestinal obstruction, intra-abdominal abscess or sepsis or the presence of most intra-abdominal fistulae. Recently, however, a successful laparoscopic resection for ileocolonic Crohn's disease including both ileal stenosis and ileovesical fistula is reported from Japan[79] suggesting that the indications are set to widen in the near future.

The Problem of Indeterminate Colitis and the Subsequent Failure of Ileoanal Pouch Procedures Because of Unsuspected Crohn's Disease

Since the introduction of ileoanal pouch procedures (IAPP) some 25 years ago there has been a constant problem with patients initially thought to have ulcerative colitis but subsequently found to have Crohn's colitis. Generally the outlook for patients who have Crohn's disease and who are treated by IAPP is poor. This poor outcome has focused attention on how to avoid the problem by careful case selection. Few surgeons have purposefully carried out IAPP in patients with known Crohn's disease although Panis and colleagues[80] do report a small series of highly selected patients who were thought to have colonic Crohn's disease. These patients had no evidence of anal, perianal or small bowel disease. In these very carefully selected patients approximately 50% retained their pouch long term. Very careful documentation of the histological material in these patients would seem important before conclusions are drawn concerning the outcome in this series as it is, of course, possible that some of these patients actually had ulcerative colitis.

Several series report an incidence of Crohn's disease subsequently discovered in patients who are initially believed to have ulcerative colitis before IAPP was performed. The incidence of undetected Crohn's colitis ranges from 3 to 7%.[81-83] Clearly patients with clinical or radiological evidence of small bowel disease or else perianal disease should be considered very carefully before IAPP is considered. The idea that a preliminary colectomy prior to IAPP might safeguard against inadvertent IAPP in patients with Crohn's colitis is attractive. Unfortunately this is not the case and several series report patients who had been treated by preliminary colectomy and then subsequently IAPP but eventually were diagnosed as suffering from Crohn's disease.[84] In patients who have had a preliminary colectomy, it may be difficult to differentiate histologically between Crohn's proctitis and defunctioned proctitis in the rectal stump.

A further group of patients who require very careful selection prior to IAPP are those with indeterminate colitis.[15,85] Up to 15% of patients with idiopathic colitis fall into this category and it is likely to be a diagnosis made especially when the colitis is very active and therefore the more characteristic features of either ulcerative or Crohn's colitis are obscured.[15] Some reports concerning the outcome of indeterminate colitis are encouraging. Pezim et al.[86] report the outcome of 25 patients with indeterminate colitis having undergone an IAPP. At 3 years of follow-up, the failure rate was low. Similarly Wells and colleagues[87] reported 16 patients with indeterminate colitis followed-up for a median of 10 years. During this time the probable diagnosis changed from indeterminate colitis to ulcerative colitis in three patients (18%) and to Crohn's colitis in one patient.6%). However, a more recent study from the Lahey Clinic[88] suggests that whereas patients with a definite diagnosis of ulcerative colitis prior to IAPP have their diagnosis revised to Crohn's colitis in only 3%, those initially considered to have indeterminate colitis had their diagnosis revised to Crohn's colitis in 13% of cases. It is therefore important to explain to those patients with indeterminate colitis that there may be an increased risk of subsequent reclassification as Crohn's disease following IAPP.

Summary

This chapter summarises the indications for surgery in patients with colonic Crohn's disease. Although the majority of patients with Crohn's disease require colectomy for failed medical treatment or acute colitis it is helpful to consider some of the less well-known indications. Following on from this the objectives of combining symptom relief with a good functional result and low recurrence rate are discussed. The prospects of laparoscopic resection for Crohn's disease of the colon look exciting for the future. Finally Crohn's colitis is an area of surgery where very careful discussion with the patient prior to operation is essential and done optimally can be richly rewarding for both patient and surgeon alike.

References

1. Janowitz HD (1975) Problems in Crohn's disease, evaluation of the results of surgical treatment. J Chronic Dis 28:63–66.
2. Elliott PR, Ritchie JK, Lennard-Jones JE (1985) Prognosis of colonic Crohn's disease. Br Med J 291:178.
3. Andrews HA, Lewis P, Allan RN (1989) Prognosis after surgery for colonic Crohn's disease. Br J Surg 76:1184–1190.
4. Keighley MRB, Allan RN (1986) Current status and influence of operation on perianal Crohn's disease. Int J Colorectal Dis 1:104–107.
5. Allan A, Keighley MRB (1988) Management of perianal Crohn's disease. World J Surg 12:198–202.
6. Connell WR, Sheffield JR, Kamm MA, Ritchie JK, Hawley PR, Lennard-Jones JE (1994) Lower gastrointestinal malignancy in Crohn's disease. Gut 35:347–352.
7. Farmer RG, Hawk WA, Turnbull RB (1975) Clinical patterns in Crohn's disease : a statistical study of 615 cases. Gastroenterology 68:627.
8. Greenstein AJ, Kark AE, Dreiling DA (1975) Crohn's disease of the colon: toxic dilatation of the colon in Crohn's colitis. Am J Gastroenterol 63:117.
9. Grieco MB, Bordan DL, Geiss AC, Beil AR (1983) Toxic megacolon complicating Crohn's colitis. Ann Surg 197:179–182.
10. Buzzard AJ, Baker WNW, Needham PRG, Warren RE (1974) Acute toxic dilatation of the colon in Crohn's colitis. Gut 15:416–419.

11. Goligher JC, Koffman DC, McDombal FT (1970) Surgical treatment of severe attack of ulcerative colitis with special reference to the advantage of early operation. Br Med J iv:703–704.

12. Travis S, Farrant JM, Ricketts C, Nolan DJ, Mortensen NJMcC, Kettlewell MGW (1996) Predicting outcome in severe ulcerative colitis. Gut 38:905–910.

13. Truelove SC, Jewell DP (1974) Intensive intravenous regimen for severe attacks of ulcerative colitis. Lancet I:1067–1070.

14. Lichtinger S, Present DH, Kornbluth A (1994) Cyclosporin in severe ulcerative colitis refractory to steroid therapy. N Engl. J Med 330:1841–1845.

15. Price AB (1978) Overlap in the spectrum of non-specific inflammatory bowel disease: "colitis indeterminate". J Clin Pathol 31:567–577.

16. Flint G, Strauss R, Platt N, Wise L (1997) Ileorectal anastomosis in patients with Crohn's disease of the colon. Gut 18:236–239.

17. Fernandez-Herliky L (1959) The articular manifestation of chronic ulcerative colitis: an analysis of 555 cases. N Engl J Med 261:259–263.

18. Sanitz AM, Greenberg MS (1951) Skin lesions in association with colitis. Gastroenterology 19:476–479.

19. Gelernt IM, Kreel I (1976) Pyoderma gangrenosum in ulcerative colitis: prevention of the gangrenous component. Mt Sinai J Med 43:467–470.

20. Greenstein AJ, Janowitz MD, Sachar DB (1976) The extraintestinal complications of Crohn's disease and ulcerative colitis. a study of 700 patients. Medicine 55:401–412.

21. Billson FA, DeDombal FT, Wilkinson G, Goligher JC (1967) Ocular complications of ulcerative colitis. Gut 8:102–106.

22. Maratka Z, Nedbal J (1964) Urolithiasis as a complication of the surgical treatment of ulcerative colitis. Gut 5:216–217.

23. Verbanck J, Lamiere N, Preet M, Pingoin A, Elewnort A, Barbier F (1979) Renal amyloidosis as a complication of Crohn's disease. Acta Clin Belg 34:6–13.

24. Werther JL, Shapira A Rubenstein O, Janowitz HD (1960) Amyloidosis in regional enteritis Am J Med 29:416–423.

25. Shorvon PJ (1997) Amyloidosis and inflammatory bowel disease. Am J Dig Dis 22:209–213.

26. Fitchen JH (1975) Amyloidosis and granulomatous ileocolitis. N Engl J Med 292:352–353.

27. Altman AR, Meltz CR, Janowitz D (1979) Autoimmune haemolytic anaemia in ulcerative colitis. Dig Dis Sci 24:282–285.

28. Kirshner BS, Klick JR, Kalman SS (1981) Reversal of growth retardation in Crohn's disease emphasising oral nutritional restitution. Gastroenterology 80:10–11.

29. Sugita A, Kogani K, Harada H, Yamazati Y, Fukushima T, Shimada H (1995) Surgery for Crohn's anal fistula. J Gastroenterol 30:143–146.

30. Harper PH, Kettlewell MGW, Lee ECG (1982) The effect of split ileostomy on perianal Crohn's disease. Br J Surg 69:608–610.

31. Nordgren S, Fasth S, Hulten L (1992) Anal fistulas, incidence and outcome of surgical treatment. Int J Colorectal Dis 7:214–218.

32. Glotzer DJ (1995) Surgical therapy for Crohn's disease. Gastroenterol Clin North Am 24:577–596.

33. Higgins CS, Keighley MRB, Allan RN (1981) Impact of pre-operative weight loss on post-operative morbidity. J R Soc Med 74:571–575.

34. Irving MH (1990) The management of surgical complications of Crohn's disease abscess and fistula. In: Allan RN, Keighley MRB, Alexander-Williams J, Hawkin C (eds) Inflammatory bowel disease. Churchill. Livingstone, Edinburgh, pp 489–500.

35. Mullen JL, Hargrove WC, Dudricks ST, Fitts WT, Rosata EF (1978) Ten year experience with iv hyperalimentation and parenteral nutrition. Ann Surg 187:523–529.

36. Rombeau JL, Bardot IE, Williamson CE, Mullen JL (1982) Pre–operative TPN and surgical outcome in patients with inflammatory bowel disease. Am J Surg 143:134–143.

37. Buzby GP (1991) Perioperative total parenteral nutrition in surgical patients. N Engl J Med 325:525.

38. Detsky AS (1991) Perioperative total parenteral nutrition in surgical patients. N Engl J Med 325:573.

39. Andrews HA, Keighley MRB, Alexander-Williams J, Allan RN (1991) Strategy for management of distal ileal Crohn's disease. Br J Surg 78:679–682.

40. Zelas P, Jagelman DG (1980) Loop ileostomy in the management of Crohn's colitis in the debiltated patient. Ann Surg 191:164–168.

41. Harper PH, Truelove SC, Lee ECG, Kettlewell MGW, Jewell DP (1983) Split ileostomy and ileostomy for Crohn's disease of the colon: a 20-year survey. Gut 24:106–113.

42. Alexander-Williams J (1974) Loop ileostomy and colostomy for faecal diversion. Ann R Coll Surg Engl 54:141–148.

43. Lee ECG (1975) Split ileostomy in the treatment of Crohn's disease of the colon. Ann R Coll Surg Engl 56:94–102.
44. Oberhelman HA (1976) The effect of intestinal diversion by ileostomy on Crohn's disease of the colon. In: Weterman IT, Pena AS, Booth CC (eds) The management of Crohn's disease. Excerpta Medica, Amsterdam, pp 216–219.
45. Allan A, Andrews H, Hilton CJ, Keighley MRB, Allan RN, Alexander-Williams J (1989) Segmental colectomy is an appropriate operation for short skip lesions due to Crohn's disease in the colon. World J Surg 13:611–616.
46. Ambrose NS, Keighley MRB, Alexander-Williams J, Allan RN (1984) Clinical impact of colectomy and ileo-rectal anastomosis in the management of Crohn's disease. Gut 25:223–227.
47. Keighley MRB, Buchmann P, Lee JR (1982) Assessment of anorectal function in selection of patients for ileo-rectal anastomosis in Crohn's colitis. Gut 23:102–107.
48. Lefton HB, Farmer RG, Fazio V (1975) Ileorectal anastomosis for Crohn's disease of the colon. Gastroenterology 69:612–617.
49. Allan RN, Steinberg DM, Alexander-Williams J, Cook WT (1977) Crohn's disease involving the colon: an audit of clinical management. Gastroenterology 73:723–732.
50. Buckmann P, Weterman IT, Keighley MRB, Pena AS, Allan RN, Alexander-Williams J (1981) The prognosis of ileo–rectal anastomosis in Crohn's disease. Br J Surg 68:7–10.
51. Cooper JC, Jones D, Williams NS (1986) Outcome of colectomy and ileorectal anastomosis in Crohn's disease. Ann R Coll Surg Engl 68:279–282.
52. Scammell BE, Keighley MRB (1985) Delayed perineal wound healing after proctectomy for Crohn's colitis. Br J Surg 73:150–152.
53. Fazio VW, Floriano-Marcettis J, Church JM et al. (1996) Effect of resection margins on the recurrence of Crohn's disease in the small bowel. Ann Surg 224:563–573.
54. Ihasz M, Batorfi I, Balint A et al. (1995) Surgical relations of Crohn's disease and the frequency of recurrence. Acta Chir Hung 35:63–75.
55. Post S, Herfarth, Böhm E et al. (1996) The impact of disease pattern, surgical management and individual surgeons on the risk for relaparotomy for recurrent Crohn's disease. Ann Surg 223:253–260.
56. Goldberg PA, Wright JP, Gerber M, Classen R (1993) Incidence of surgical resection for Crohn's disease. Dis Colon Rectum 36:736–739.
57. D'Haens. GR, Rutgeerts P (1994) Post-operative recurrence of Crohn's disease, pathogenesis and prevention. Acta Gastroenterol Belg 57:311–313.
58. Aeberhard P, Berchtold W, Riedtmann HJ, Stadelman G (1996) Surgical recurrence of perforating and non-perforating Crohn's disease. Dis Colon Rectum 39:80–87.
59. Raab Y, Bergströn R, Ejerblad J, Graf W, Pahlman L (1996) Factors influencing recurrence in Crohn's disease. Dis Colon Rectum 39:918–925.
60. Sachar DB (1996) Patterns of postoperative recurrence in fistulizing and stenotic Crohn's disease. Clin Gastroenterol 22:114–116.
61. Holzheimer RG, Molloy RG, Witman DH (1995) Post-operative complications predict recurrence of Crohn's disease. Eur J Surg 161:129–135.
62. Smedh K, Olaison G, Nystrom PO, Sjondahl R (1993) Intra-operative enteroscopy in Crohn's disease. Br J Surg 80:897–900.
63. Shivananda S, Mordijk ML, Pena AS, Mayberry JF (1989) Crohn's disease, risk of recurrence and re-operation in a defined population. Gut 30:990–998.
64. Souftly A, Myren J, Clamp SE, Bouchier IA, Watkinson G, da Dombal FT (1988) Affecting recurrence after surgery for Crohn's disease. Scand J Gastroenterolgy (Suppl) 144:31–34.
65. Rutgeerts P, Geboes K, Vantrappen G, Kerremans R, Coenegrachts J L, Coremans G (1984) Natural history of recurrent Crohn's disease at the ileocaecal anastomosis after curative surgery. Gut 25:665–672.
66. Rutgeerts, Geboes K, Vantrappen G, Beyls J, Kerremans R, Hiele M (1990) Predictability of the post-operative course of Crohn's disease. Gastroenterology 99:956–963.
67. Pallona , Boirivant M, Stazi MA, Coslintino R, Prentera C, Torsoli A (1992) Analysis of clinical course of post-operative recurrence in Crohn's disease of the distal ileum. Dig Dis Sci 37:215–219.
68. Tytgat GNJ, Ulder CJ, Brummelkemp WH (1988) Endoscopic lesions in Crohn's disease early after ileo-caecal resection. Endoscopy 20:260–262.
69. Brignola C, Cottone M, Pena A, Italian Co-operative Study Group (1985) Mesalamine in the prevention of endoscopic recurrence after intestinal resection for Crohn's disease. Gastroenterology 108:345–349.
70. Caprilli R, Corrao G, Taddei G, Torselli F, Torchio P, Viscido A, Gruppo Italiano per lo Studio Del Colon E Del Retto (1996) Prognostic factors for post-operative recurrence of Crohn's disease. Dis Colon Rectum 39:335–341.

71. McLeod RS, Wolff BG, Steinhart AM et al (1995) Prophylactic mesalamine treatment decreases post-operative recurrence of Crohn's disease. Gastroenterology 109:404–413.

72. Cottone M, Rosselli M, Orlando A (1994) Smoking habits and recurrence in Crohn's disease. Gastroenterology 106:643–648.

73. Ritchie JK (1996) The results of surgery for large bowel Crohn's disease. Ann R Coll Surg Engl 72:155–157.

74. Scammell BE, Ambrose NS, Alexander-Williams J, Allan RN, Keighley MRB (1985) Recurrent small bowel Crohn's disease is more frequent after subtotal colectomy and ileorectal anastomosis than proctocolectomy. Dis Colon Rectum 28:770–771.

75. Wettergren A, Christiansen J (1991) Risk of recurrence and re-operation after resection for ileo-colic Crohn's disease. Scand J Gastroenterol 26:1319–1322.

76. Cameron JL, Hamilton SR, Coleman J, Sitzmann JV. Bayless TM (1992) Patterns of ileal recurrence in Crohn's disease. a prospective randomised study. Ann Surg 215:546–551.

77. Scott NA, Sueling HM, Hughes LE (1995) Anastomotic configuration does not affect recurrence of Crohn's disease after ileo-colonic resection. Int J Colorectal Dis 10:67–69.

78. Ludwig KA, Milsom JW, Church JM, Fazio VW (1996) Preliminary experience with laparoscopic intestinal surgery for Crohn's disease. Am J Surg 171:52–56.

79. Sizawa H, Hibi T, Ohishi T et al. (1996) Laparoscopic assisted ileocaecal resection for Crohn's disease associated with intestinal stenosis and ileovesical fistula. J Gastroenterol 31:425–430.

80. Panis Y, Popard B, Nemeth J, Lavergne A, Heutofeville P, Valleur P (1996) Ileal pouch anal anastomosis for Crohn's disease. Lancet 347:854–857.

81. Deutche A, McLeod RS, Cullen J, Cohen Z (1991) Results of the pelvic pouch procedure in patients with Crohn's disease. Dis Colon Rectum 34:475–477.

82. Nicholls RJ (1987) Restorative proctolectomy with various tyres of reservoir. World J Surg 11:751–762.

83. Hymen HH, Fazio VW, Tuckson WB, Lavery IC (1991) The consequences of ileal pouch-anal anastomosis for Crohn's disease. Dis Colon Rectum 34:653–657.

84. Poppen B, Svenberg T, Bark T (1992) Colectomy: proctomucosectomy with S pouch: operative procedures complications and functional outcome in 69 consective patients. Dis Colon Rectum 32:40–47.

85. Price AB (1996) Indeterminate colitis; broadening the prospective. Curr Diagn Pathol 3:35–44.

86. Pezim ME, Pemberton JH, Beart KW (1989) outcome of "indeterminate colitis" following ileal pouch-anal anastomosis. Dis Colon Rectum 32:653–658.

87. Wells AD, McMillan I, Price AB, Ritchie JK, Nicholls RJ (1991) Natural history of indeterminate colitis. Br J Surg 78:179–181.

88. Marcellow PW, Shoetz DJ, Roberts PL et al. (1996) Evolutionary changes in pathologic diagnosis following the ileoanal pouch procedure. Int J Colorectal Dis 1996:11:145.

5 Imaging of the Anal Canal and Rectum

D.M. Gold and W. A. Kmiot

Prior to 1989 the only method of anal sphincter mapping was by utilising a painful technique of electromyography. Recently, new radiological techniques for anal sphincter imaging have evolved that include endoanal ultrasound and magnetic resonance imaging (with surface and endoluminal coils). These techniques are now available to provide information on anal sphincter anatomy in patients with traumatic or idiopathic faecal incontinence, anorectal sepsis and anorectal malignancy.

Endoanal/Endorectal Ultrasound

Methods and Technique

The most commonly used ultrasound endoprobe for anal sphincter imaging is the Bruel and Kjaer, Type 1850, rotating scanner (Fig. 5.1a,b), first described by Frentzel-Beyme[1] in 1982 for imaging the prostate gland. Using the same probe, Beynon et al.[2] characterised endosonography of the normal colon and rectum and demonstrated the accuracy of this technique in staging of rectal carcinoma.

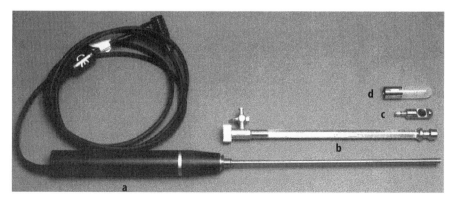

Fig. 5.1a–d. The unassembled probe. **a** The handle housing the motor, attached to the rotating rod. **b** The rectal tube which fits over the rod. Water is injected with a syringe via the nozzle at the base of the tube. **c** The 10-MHz transducer which fits a tip of the rotating rod. **d** The TPX plastic cone which fits over the transducer.

Prior to introduction of endoanal ultrasound, sphincter defects were mapped using electrophysiological techniques. The accuracy of endoanal ultrasound has been correlated with electromyography and proven to be accurate in the determination of sphincter defects.[3–5] This has led to the routine use of endoanal ultrasound in the investigation of faecal incontinence following obstetric damage, trauma or iatrogenic sphincter division.[6]

In order to to image the anal sphincters and protect the transducer (Fig. 5.1c) from direct tissue contact a solid plastic cone (Fig. 5.1d) was introduced.[7] This innovation generated much interest and the sonographic appearance of the anal sphincters were correlated with in vivo and in vitro anatomy.[8] This work identified the subepithelium, internal sphincter, longitudinal muscle, and external sphincter and demonstrated important differences in the sphincter configuration of male and female anal canals.

Modern anal endosonographic practice uses a high-frequency 10-MHz crystal (Fig. 5.1c) which, by decreasing the depth of penetration of the sound wave, gives far greater image resolution, providing a lateral resolution of 0.05 mm and a slice thickness of 0.8 mm.

A rotating endoprobe provides 360° images of the anal sphincters and is protected from the tissues of the anal canal by a solid plastic cone (Fig. 5.1d), filled with degassed (boiled and cooled) tap-water to maintain acoustic coupling. The cone is then covered with a sonolucent gel and a condom to prevent contamination. More gel is applied to the outside of the condom and the probe is then inserted into the canal. Patients are scanned in either the left lateral position or in some cases where the anal canal is short, lying prone, which improves the symmetry of the scanned image.[9]

Insertion of the probe beyond the anal canal and into the rectum is easily recognised by loss of acoustic coupling and the development of reverberation echoes as well as loss of the "circular" internal sphincter as it becomes the more irregular circular muscle layer of the rectum. The probe is orientated so that the anterior structures in the anal canal are uppermost on the screen. Abnormalities of the anal sphincters are described like that of a 12-hour clock-face with 12 o'clock anterior, i.e. uppermost in the image.

Normal Endosonographic Anatomy

The normal endosonographic appearance of the anal canal is a four-layered structure consisting of a hyperchoic subepithelium, hypoechoic internal sphincter, hyperechoic longitudinal muscle and heteroechoic external sphincter (Fig. 5.2).

Sphincter Defects

Anal incontinence for gas or faeces affects up to 11% of adults. The commonest cause in healthy women is unrecognised damage to the anal sphincters during childbirth; 13% of women having their first vaginal delivery develop incontinence or urgency, and 30% have structural changes. The commonest predisposing cause of damage is the use of forceps.[10] Other recognised causes are perianal sepsis, anal surgery and non-obstetric trauma.

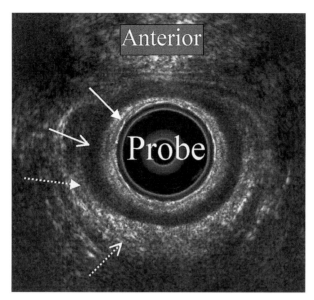

Fig. 5.2. Conventional two-dimensional endoanal ultrasound image in the transverse plane. The subepithelium (solid arrow) can be seen encircling the bright interface reflection from the outer rim of the plastic cone. The hypoechoic internal sphincter (solid open arrow) is a low reflective ring. The longitudinal muscle (dotted solid arrow) is a moderately reflective layer, within the striated texture of the external sphincter (dotted open arrow).

Confirmation of the presence of endosonographically detected sphincter defects with electromyography showed a 100% sensitivity for external sphincter defects.[3,4,11,12] It also provided information on damage to the internal sphincter. The accuracy of determining sphincter defects has also been confirmed histologically[5,13] with up to 100% sensitivity and specificity for external sphincter defects and 100% sensitivity and 95.5% specificity for internal sphincter defects.

The main reason for performing endoanal ultrasound in incontinence is to distinguish idiopathic incontinence from sphincter defects and to provide accurate anatomical information of sphincter anatomy and configuration prior to surgical repair (Fig. 5.3).[14] Numerous studies have shown the benefit of sphincter repair with functional improvement in 76–93% of cases and a postoperative increase in maximum squeeze pressure of up to 11–15 cmH$_2$O.[15-17] Outcome is further improved if postoperative sonographic assessment confirms an intact external anal sphincter (EAS) ring. One study showed 32 of 35 patients improved where the EAS was intact compared with 5 of 11 where a defect persisted.[15] There is no contraindication to sphincter repair in the elderly as functional outcome after surgery appears equal to that of younger patients.[17]

As endoanal ultrasound produces only axial images and does not give the operating surgeon any measurements as to the extent of the defect it may be that incomplete repair results from lack of appreciation of the longitudinal extent at the time of surgery. Furthermore, it has been shown that in incomplete repair the angular measurement of the remaining defect has decreased (Fig. 5.4).[18]

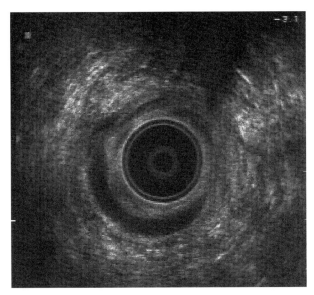

Fig. 5.3. An endoanal sonogram showing an internal sphincter defect between 4 o'clock and 9 o'clock, and an external sphincter defect between 11 o'clock and 2 o'clock.

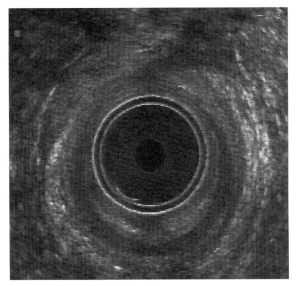

Fig. 5.4. A failed repair. An external sphincter defect still exists between 12 o'clock and 1 o'clock. (An internal sphincter defect also exists between 9 o'clock and 2 o'clock.)

Endosonography in Anal Sepsis

Anal endosonography is a sensitive technique for the demonstration of inter-sphincteric and transsphincteric fistulae and perianal collections (Fig. 5.5a,b).[19] Unfortunately, it is no more accurate than an examining finger in the accurate

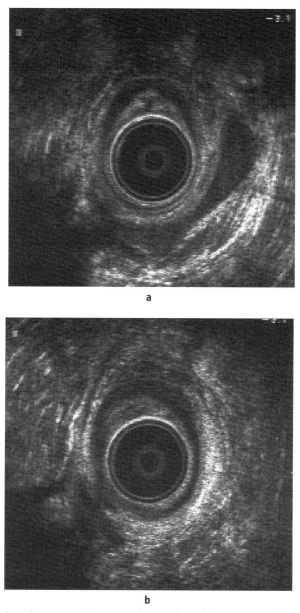

Fig. 5.5. a An endoanal sonogram showing an intersphincteric horse-shoe cavity (black) between 2 o'clock and 7 o'clock in the upper canal. **b** More distally the cavity opens into the canal at 7 o'clock and is associated with a transsphincteric track to an extrasphincteric abscess cavity.

identification of the internal fistulous opening, and is unable accurately to assess the primary and secondary tracks in suprasphincteric and supralevator fistulae owing to loss of tissue contact with the plastic cone around the transducer.[20] Furthermore, when assessing recurrent disease it is not possible to distinguish between active sepsis and fibrous scar tissue as both are hypoechoic in appearance. In complex cases the routine use of endosonography has been superseded by magnetic resonance imaging (MRI).

Malignancy

Endorectal sonography using an inflatable balloon to surround the transducer is a useful modality in determining local stage of rectal cancer and in determining sphincter involvement to aid patient selection for appropriate treatment. A prospective study of 28 patients has shown depth of invasion to be accurate in 78.5% of cases. Involvement of perirectal fat demonstrated 96% sensitivity and 76% specificity and lymph node staging 81% sensitivity and 50% specificity.[21] Technical problems in ultrasound of the rectal wall include proximity of the lesion to the anal verge, improper balloon inflation, an oblique imaging plane, a transducer gain setting that is too high and artefacts due to shadowing of air or stool, reverberation, or refraction. Sources of error in tumour staging with endorectal ultrasound include interpretation differences, endosonographer bias, tumour location, tumour stenosis, peritumoural inflammation, post-surgical changes, post-irradiation changes, haemorrhage, and pedunculated or villous tumours. Node size and appearance are not reliable indicators of lymph node involvement.[22,23]

Squamous cell carcinoma of the anal canal, although relatively rare, accounts for approximately 3% of malignant tumours affecting the large bowel. The current treatment of choice is radiotherapy with or without chemotherapy. Anal endosonography is an accurate method of asssessing these tumours and can classify the depth of the tumour invasion into four levels, UT1, confined to the epithelium; UT2, involving the internal sphincter/longitudinal muscle; UT3, involving the external sphincter or UT4, penetration through the external sphincter.[24] Endoanal ultrasonography has an accuracy of 92% against 72% for computed tomography (CT), when compared with histological findings,[25] and may act as an accurate predictor of outcome with different treatment modalities, as all T1–T2/ UT1–UT2 tumours responded completely to the initial radiotherapy with or without chemotherapy.[24,25]

Magnetic Resonance Imaging (MRI)

In vitro histological anatomy of the anal canal has been well correlated with MRI findings.[26] Initial studies of in vivo sphincter anatomy were originally performed with body coils but found that differentiation between mucosa, submucosa and internal anal sphincter was not possible.[27] These techniques have now been superseded by the incorporation of an internal coil in addition to the surface coil.

Endoanal MRI

The use of a dedicated endoanal receiving coil, with an integrated hybrid circuit encased in a Delrin (acetylhomopolymer) former was originally employed for imaging the prostate.[28] Modification of the cylindrical coil to produce a saddle geometry to encompass the anal sphincters produces high quality images. A 0.5 T (Tesla) or for superior image quality, 1.0 T magnetic field is used. T1-, T2-weighted and STIR (short tau inversion recovery) sequences are routinely employed.

Imaging of the sphincters is performed with the patient supine. The receiver coil, 9 mm in diameter and 7.5 cm in length is placed into the anorectum and held still in a clamp between the patient's legs.

MRI images of the anal canal demonstrate a higher signal from the internal anal sphincter (IAS) than the EAS in contrast to the reflections obtained from the ultrasound probe. This is thought to be related to the smooth muscle component of the internal sphincter as a similar signal is seen from the smooth muscle component of the myometrium when the uterus is scanned endovaginally. Anatomically, owing to its ability to provide multiplanar images, MRI has confirmed the shorter anterior EAS in females suggested by endoanal ultrasound and shows the EAS to be either a two- or three-part structure depending on the ability to distinguish between the superficial and subcutaneous components, which have been described to a variable degree.[29–33]

Sphincter Defects

Owing to the ability of MRI to image directly the muscle fibres of the sphincters as opposed to internal reflections within the sphincter, seen on EUS, MRI provides high-quality easily interpreted images of the anal sphincters. One prospective study has compared MR imaging of obstetric sphincter trauma with surgical findings and found 100% sensitivity for sphincter defects (Fig. 5.6).[34]

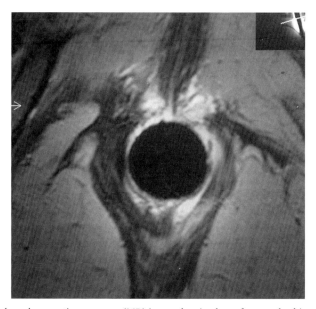

Fig. 5.6. An endoanal magnetic resonance (MR) image showing loss of external sphincter (dark grey) between 11 o'clock and 6 o'clock.

Although MR images are more easily understood by an operating surgeon the ability of endoanal sonography to detect these defects, when compared with MRI appears similar, and EUS has the advantage in that it may be used intraoperatively. MRI is unlikely to supersede ultrasound in the routine investigation of obstetric sphincter defects as it is more costly, less readily available and takes considerably longer to perform.

MRI and Anorectal Sepsis

Endoanal sonography, although valuable in the detection of localised intersphincteric abscess cavities is limited in the assessment of anorectal sepsis owing to its inability to demonstrate internal fistulous openings and to provide images above the puborectalis. It is also unable to distinguish active disease from scar tissue, both appearing black on the sonographic image.

Non-invasive MR surface coil studies in patients with complex recurrent fistulae have shown a high degree of accuracy in the determining primary and secondary fistulous tracks, in the identification of fistulous openings and suggest that MRI may demonstrate abnormalites not detected preoperatively by the examining finger.[35,36] Imaging of anorectal sepsis with MRI shows concordance with operative findings of 86% for the presence and course of the primary tracks, 91% for the presence and site of secondary extensions and 97% for the presence of horseshoeing (Fig. 5.7).[37]

The use of gadolinium-enhanced, STIR sequence MR provides high-resolution images that accurately define pus from granulation tissue and normal pelvic floor anatomy. However, as with EUS, the reduced field of view when using the endocoil

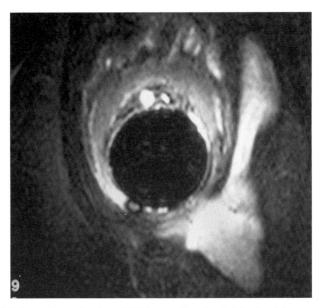

Fig. 5.7. A gadolinium-enhanced endoanal MR image. There is a bright signal from an abscess cavity at 5 o'clock with a left-sided extrasphincteric horseshoe extension.

alone may miss high supralevator tracks and surface MR views must be performed in all patients.

MRI in Malignancy

MRI has been shown to provide detailed information on the local staging of rectal carcinoma when compared with surgical findings.[34] Whether or not this provides a greater benefit over the information provided by CT has been questionable. A comparative study between endoscopic ultrasound and endocoil MRI in rectal cancer[38] showed greater accuracy with EUS in the T-staging of primary tumours (n=6), (due to the better differentiation between T1 and T2 tumours), but similar positive and negative predictive values in the detection of recurrent disease (n=15). A larger prospective study comparing surface MRI, endocoil MR and EUS[39] also found similar accuracy for depth of bowel wall penetration of rectal carcinomas but suggested that in advanced cases surface coil imaging would provide greater information about the extent of intra-abdominal spread.

Three-Dimensional Endoanal Sonography

Conventional endoanal ultrasound is limited in that it does not provide any longitudinal information on the sphincters. A system for providing multiplanar three-dimensional images has recently been developed.[40] By using a linear translational rig (to register accurate, evenly spaced longitudinal movement of the probe within the anal canal) it is possible to obtain a series of ultrasound images only 1.25 mm apart. Using a suitable three-dimensional PC-based program these images can be reconstructed into digital volumes which facilitate multiplanar slicing and accurate measurement.

This technique has been applied in the investigation of sphincter defects. A direct relationship between the radial angle of a defect and its longitudinal extent has been demonstrated in obstetric and iatrogenic trauma. This response to trauma is similar for both the internal and external sphincter and may provide an understanding of the role played by the longitudinal muscle in acting as a support for the sphincter muscles. Gender differences in external sphincter configuration have also been demonstrated with this technique, suggesting that the male anal canal is longer than the female canal, and that the external sphincter is present anteriorly for a greater proportional length (Fig. 5.8a,b).[41]

Three dimensional reconstructions of MR images are now being developed[42] but at present do not offer the image resolution of reconstructed ultrasound images.

Summary

Endoanal ultrasound and MRI represent a significant advance in the imaging and understanding of anorectal anatomy and pathology. Both modalities provide high-quality images which are reproducible and have been well validated against in vitro and surgical dissections in a small number of subjects. Endoanal ultra-

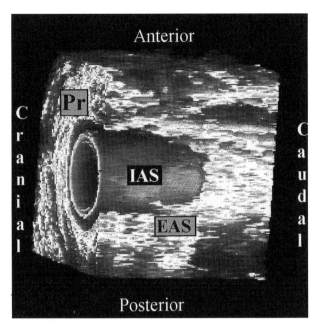

a

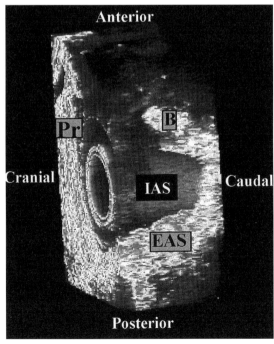

b

sound is less troublesome to the patient, cheaper, more readily available, quicker to perform and can be used intraoperatively. It should remain as the first-line investigation of all sphincter pathologies: traumatic, septic or malignant. MRI should be reserved for the more complex case as its ability to provide multiplanar images may provide greater information of relevance to clinical decision making. Three-dimensional imaging of the anal canal with ultrasound may redress the multiplanar advantages of MRI and direct comparative studies are awaited.

References

1. Frentzel-Beyme B (1982) Die transrektale prostatasonographie. Computertomogr Sonogr 2(2):58–112.
2. Beynon J, Mortensen NJ, Foy DM, Channer JL, Virjee J, Goddard P (1986) Pre-operative assessment of local invasion in rectal cancer: digital examination, endoluminal sonography or computed tomography? Br J Surg 73:1015–1017.
3. Burnett SJ, Speakman CT, Kamm MA, Bartram CI (1991) Confirmation of endosonographic detection of external anal sphincter defects by simultaneous electromyographic mapping. Br J Surg 78:448–450.
4. Law PJ, Kamm MA, Bartram CI (1990) A comparison between electromyography and anal endosonography in mapping external anal sphincter defects. Dis Colon Rectum 33:370–373.
5. Deen KI, Kumar D, Williams JG, Olliff J, Keighley MR (1993) Anal sphincter defects. Correlation between endoanal ultrasound and surgery. Ann Surg 218:201–205.
6. Deen KI, Kumar D, Williams JG, Olliff J, Keighley MR (1993) The prevalence of anal sphincter defects in faecal incontinence: a prospective endosonic study. Gut 34:685–688.
7. Law PJ, Bartram CI (1989) Anal endosonography: technique and normal anatomy. Gastrointest Radiol 14:349–353.
8. Sultan AH, Nicholls RJ, Kamm MA, Hudson CN, Beynon J, Bartram CI (1993) Anal endosonography and correlation with in vitro and in vivo anatomy. Br J Surg 80:508–511.
9. Cavaye DM, Tabbara MR, Kopchok GE, Laas TE, Cormier F, White RA (1991) A new technique for intraluminal hollow organ imaging: three-dimensional ultrasound. J Laparoendosc Surg 1:259–268.
10. Kamm MA (1994) Obstetric damage and faecal incontinence. Lancet 344:730–733.
11. Sorensen M, Nielsen MB, Pedersen JF, Christiansen J (1994) Electromyography of the internal anal sphincter performed under endosonographic guidance. Description of a new method. Dis Colon Rectum 37:138–143
12. Tjandra JJ, Milsom JW, Schroeder T, Fazio VW (1993) Endoluminal ultrasound is preferable to electromyography in mapping anal sphincteric defects. Dis Colon Rectum 36:689–692.
13. Sultan AH, Kamm MA, Talbot IC, Nicholls RJ, Bartram CI (1994) Anal endosonography for identifying external sphincter defects confirmed histologically.Br J Surg 81:463–465.
14. Nielsen MB, Hauge C, Pedersen JF, Christiansen J (1993) Endosonographic evaluation of patients with anal incontinence: findings and influence on surgical management. AJR 160:771–775.
15. Engel AF, Kamm MA, Sultan AH, Bartram CI, Nicholls RJ (1994) Anterior anal sphincter repair in patients with obstetric trauma. Br J Surg 81:1231–1234.
16. Fleshman JW, Peters WR, Shemesh EI, Fry RD, Kodner IJ (1991) Anal sphincter reconstruction: anterior overlapping muscle repair. Dis Colon Rectum 34:739–743.

◀ **Fig. 5.8. a** A three-dimensional representation of the male anal canal. The puborectalis (Pr) at the proximal aspect of the canal is difficult to distinguish from the external anal sphincter (EAS). The EAS is present along the full length of the canal anteriorly. The internal anal sphincter (IAS) terminates approximately in the mid-canal level. The subcutaneous external sphincter is longer in this patient than the female example. **b** A three-dimensional representation of the female anal canal. The left side of the U-shaped puborectalis (Pr) can be seen at the proximal end of the canal. The right aspect of the IAS terminates approximately two-thirds the way down the canal. The EAS is seen to form an anterior ring just prior to the termination of the IAS and continues as the subcutaneous external sphincter. The bulbospongiosus muscle (B) is anterior to the external anal sphincter.

17. Simmang C, Birnbaum EH, Kodner IJ, Fry RD, Fleshman JW (1994) Anal sphincter reconstruction in the elderly: does advancing age affect outcome? Dis Colon Rectum 37:1065–1069.
18. Nielsen MB, Dammegaard L, Pedersen JF (1994) Endosonographic assessment of the anal sphincter after surgical reconstruction. Dis Colon Rectum 37:434–438.
19. Law PJ, Talbot RW, Bartram CI, Northover JM (1989) Anal endosonography in the evaluation of perianal sepsis and fistula in ano. Br J Surg 76:752–755.
20. Choen S, Burnett S, Bartram CI, Nicholls RJ (1991)Comparison between anal endosonography and digital examination in the evaluation of anal fistulae. Br J Surg 78:445–447.
21. Jayet C, Cuttat JF, Wassmer FA, Suter M (1994) [Endorectal ultrasound of rectal cancers]. Helv Chir Acta 60:687–689.
22. Akasu T, Sugihara K, Moriya Y, Fujita S (1997) Limitations and pitfalls of transrectal staging of rectal cancer. Dis Colon Rectum 40:S10–S15.
23. Kruskal JB, Kane RA, Sentovich SM, Longmaid HE (1997) Pitfalls and sources of error in staging rectal cancer with endorectal us. Radiographics 17:609–626.
24. Goldman S, Norming U, Svensson C, Glimelius B (1991) Transanorectal ultrasonography in the staging of anal epidermoid carcinoma. Int J Colorectal Dis 6:152–157.
25. Giovannini M, Seitz JF, Sfedj D, Houvenaeghel G, Delpero JR (1992) [Transanorectal ultrasonography in the evaluation of extension and the monitoring of epidermoid cancers of the anus treated by radiation or chemotherapy]. Gastroenterol Clin Biol 16:994–998.
26. Van Beers BE, Kartheuser A, Delos MA, Grandin C, Detry R, Jamart J, Pringot J (1996) MRI of the anal canal: correlation with histologic examination. Magn Reson Imaging 14:151–156.
27. Schafer A, Enck P, Furst G, Kahn T, Frieling T, Lubke HJ (1994) Anatomy of the anal sphincters. Comparison of anal endosonography to magnetic resonance imaging. Dis Colon Rectum 37:777–781.
28. Schnall MD, Lenkinski RE, Pollack HM, Imai Y, Kressel HY (1989) Prostate MR imaging with an endorectal surface coil. Radiology 172:570–574.
29. deSouza NM, Puni R, Gilderdale DJ, Bydder GM (1995) Magnetic resonance imaging of the anal sphincter using an internal coil. Magn Reson Q 11:45–56.
30. deSouza NM, Puni R, Kmiot WA, Bartram CI, Hall AS, Bydder GM (1995) MRI of the anal sphincter. J Comput Assist Tomogr 19:745–751.
31. Hussain SM, Stoker J, Zwamborn AW, Den Hollander JC, Kuiper JW, Entius CA, Lameris JS (1996) Endoanal MRI of the anal sphincter complex: correlation with cross-sectional anatomy and histology. J Anat 189:677–682.
32. deSouza NM, Kmiot WA, Puni R, Hall AS, Burl M, Bartram CI, Bydder (1995) GM. High resolution magnetic resonance imaging of the anal sphincter using an internal coil. Gut 37:284–287.
33. Sultan AH, Kamm MA, Hudson CN, Nicholls JR, Bartram CI (1994) Endosonography of the anal sphincters: normal anatomy and comparison with manometry. Clin Radiol 49:368–374.
34. deSouza NM, Hall AS, Puni R, Gilderdale DJ, Young IR, Kmiot WA (1996) High resolution magnetic resonance imaging of the anal sphincter using a dedicated endoanal coil. Comparison of magnetic resonance imaging with surgical findings. Dis Colon Rectum 39:926–934.
35. Lunniss PJ, Armstrong P, Barker PG, Reznek RH, Phillips RK (1992) Magnetic resonance imaging of anal fistulae. Lancet 340:394–396.
36. Van Beers B, Grandin C, Kartheuser A et al. (1994) MRI of complicated anal fistulae: comparison with digital examination. J Comput Assist Tomogr 18:87–90.
37. Barker PG, Lunniss PJ, Armstrong P, Reznek RH, Cottam K, Phillips RK (1994) Magnetic resonance imaging of fistula-in-ano: technique, interpretation and accuracy. Clin Radiol 49:7–13.
38. Meyenberger C, Huch Boni RA, Bertschinger P, Zala GF, Klotz HP, Krestin GP (1995) Endoscopic ultrasound and endorectal magnetic resonance imaging: a prospective, comparative study for preoperative staging and follow-up of rectal cancer. Endoscopy 27:469–479.
39. Joosten FB, Jansen JB, Joosten HJ, Rosenbusch G (1995) Staging of rectal carcinoma using MR double surface coil, MR endorectal coil, and intrarectal ultrasound: correlation with histopathologic findings. J Comput Assist Tomogr 19:752–758.
40. Gold DM, Bartram CI, Halligan S et al. (1998) Three-dimensional endoanal ultrasound: a new technique. Gut 42 (Suppl):abstract.
41. Gold DM, Bartram CI, Halligan S, Humphries KN, Kamm MA, Kmiot WA (1999)Three-dimensional endoanal sonography in assessing anal canal injury. Br J Surg (in press).
42. Halligan S (1998) Imaging fistula-in-ano. Clin Radiol 53(2):85–95.

6 Transanal Endoscopic Microsurgery

T.A. Cook and N.J. McC. Mortensen

Introduction

Whilst the majority of small rectal adenomas are amenable to colonoscopic removal, the management of large adenomas and early cancers of the rectum is less well defined. To date options for therapy have included snare polypectomy via the colonoscope, per anal excision of the tumour, muscle-splitting perineal operations in order to perform local excision, and classical anterior resection or abdominoperineal excision of the rectum.

In recent years minimal access surgery has gained widespread acceptance and has become the standard operation for procedures such as laparoscopic cholecystectomy. It has many potential advantages including reduced postoperative pain and decreased length of hospitalisation. Transanal endoscopic microsurgery (TEM) was first described by Buess et al.[1] in 1984 and has been developed along the same lines. It extends the boundaries of transanal surgery and avoids sphincter disruption, major pelvic dissection or unnecessary resection of the rectum. Adenomas and properly selected carcinomas located up to 20 cm from the anal verge may be removed by a mucosal or full-thickness dissection followed by direct suture of the defect.

Historical Aspects

Prior to the introduction of TEM a number of different procedures were used for the removal of large rectal adenomas (Table 6.1). Anterior resection or abdominoperineal excision of the rectum (APER) have been performed but these involve major pelvic dissection with concurrent risk to the pelvic nerves. Operative mortality for anterior resection and APER ranges from 1 to 7%[2-5] and is increased in patients over the age of 70 years.[6] Fifteen per cent of patients are rendered impotent by APER and 10% have ejaculatory dysfunction.[7] Bladder dysfunction is also common with around one-third experiencing retention of urine, often requiring surgery.[8,9] Additionally those undergoing APER are condemned to a life with a permanent stoma with its attendant mechanical and psychological problems.

Attempts to manage large rectal adenomas with less invasive procedures are not new. Posterior or perineal approaches such the Kraske or Mason techniques have been developed. The Kraske approach was first described at the end of the

Table 6.1. Techniques used for excision of villous adenomas

Abdominal procedures
Anterior resection and stapled anastomosis
Abdominoperineal excision of rectum
Local procedures
Kraske technique
Mason procedure
Colonoscopic polypectomy
Transanal resection using urological resectoscope
Laser ablation
Rectal mucosectomy
Parks's per anal excision
Transanal endoscopic microsurgery

nineteenth century[10] and involves a posterior midline incision with removal of the coccyx and sometimes part of the sacrum. The rectum is approached either through or above the levators. Lymph nodes may be sampled but the procedure is associated with a high complication rate, particularly fistulae, which may occur in 21% of patients.[11,12] The Mason technique was popularised in the late 1960s.[13] This involves a parasacral incision, careful identification of the sphincters, which are divided in order to gain access to the rectum. Despite no problems with continence in Mason's original series there has been increased concern over the past few years regarding the long-term effects of sphincter disruption on continence. Additionally patients were subjected to a perineal wound that frequently took a long time to heal. These complications have led to both the Kraske and Mason techniques being superseded by anterior resection using staplers.

The advent of endoscopy led to the development of snare polypectomy. Although suitable for small, particularly pedunculated, polyps, there is an increased risk of perforation with polypectomy for larger polyps because in order to include the full circumference of the polyp more bowel wall is drawn into the snare. Large series suggest polypectomy is associated with an overall complication rate of between 1 and 2%.[14,15] Haemorrhage from the polypectomy site is the main complication but perforation represents about one-third of complications seen. A potential method of reducing the risk of perforation is to artificially raise the polyp from the bowel wall by submucosal injection of hypertonic saline with adrenaline(Fig. 6.1).[16] Alternatively the polyp can be removed in a piecemeal fashion but whilst this may reduce the risk of perforation, it is difficult to determine the depth of invasion of small carcinomas that are seen in a proportion of these polyps from the multiple fragments and recurrence rates are high.[17]

Transanal resection of large rectal adenomas has also been advocated. A resectoscope adapted from urological equipment is used to resect the tumour.[12,18,19] This also has the problems associated with piecemeal removal of tumour but is certainly useful in palliation of rectal carcinomas.

Nd.YAG and argon lasers have been used in the treatment of large rectosigmoid adenomas.[20,21] Although the complication rate is low, the recurrence rate is high. Laser therapy is usually time-consuming and may involve repeated trips to hospital for treatment, albeit on an out-patient basis. Furthermore, laser treatment does not provide any tissue for histological analysis. Since the risk of the lesion containing a focus of invasive carcinoma is around 20% and because larger lesions carry an even greater risk, laser treatment is probably confined to patients who are not fit enough to undergo a general anaesthetic.

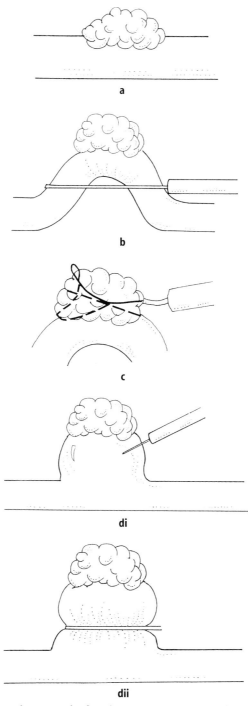

Fig. 6.1. Techniques for polypectomy for flat adenoma **a. b** Direct removal can be attempted but the bowel wall is at risk of being drawn into the snare. **c** Piecemeal excision overcomes this problem but does not permit assessment of depth of invasion of incidental carcinomas. Alternatively, hypertonic saline may be injected into the submucosal tissue **di** prior to removal **dii**

Rectal mucosectomy is a technique developed from restorative proctocolectomy and involves the complete removal of the distal rectal mucosa.[22] The procedure is based on the principle that the submucosal plane is readily distensible and the mucosa of the middle and upper rectum can be mobilised and sutured to the dentate line without tension. It has been suggested that the rectal mucosa in patients with large villous lesions might be susceptible to a field change[23] and the procedure therefore has the theoretical advantage of removing a complete ring of mucosa. A Lone Star self-retaining retractor provides exposure to the anal canal and lower rectum with minimal anal dilatation. The procedure is technically demanding and familiarity with restorative proctocolectomy and mucosectomy is an advantage. It is particularly useful in the management of large circumferential adenomas but accurate preoperative assessment to exclude elements of invasion is mandatory.

Despite the development of these various methods of local excision over the past 25 years Parks's technique[24] of per anal removal of the lesion has become the mainstay of local treatment for adenomas in the lower rectum. Per anal retractors provide good views of the anal canal and lower rectum and allow access to the tumour under direct vision. Injection of 1:200,000 adrenaline into the submucosal plane facilitates dissection although full thickness dissections can be performed if the risk of cancer is high. However, the procedure does have its limitations in that part of the luminal circumference is blocked by the retractor, and the rectum beyond the end of the retractor collapses, which may obscure the view of the proximal margin of the lesion. Consequently the procedure is suitable only for lesions in the lower rectum. Comparison of the results of this technique and TEM will be discussed later.

Equipment for TEM

The equipment that is now used for TEM has been developed by Buess's group in Germany with the assistance of the Woolf company.[25,26] Continuous evaluation and redevelopment has resulted in specific instruments dedicated for use in TEM (Fig. 6.2).

Sigmoidoscope

The operating field is viewed through a rigid sigmoidoscope with a diameter of 40 mm, which is available in two lengths, 12 and 20 cm. The sigmoidoscope has an obturator and is inserted into the rectum in a similar manner to a standard instrument. A glass window is then attached to the end and manual air insufflation allows the tumour to be visualised. Once in the optimum position, the sigmoidoscope may be locked in place with a Martin arm – a double ball and socket joint support arm connected to the operating table. This device must be within the sterile field to allow the frequent repositioning of the sigmoidoscope that is necessary during the operation. Once fixed in position the glass window is replaced by an airtight faceplate containing four ports that are sealed with rubber sleeves and provide access for the instruments.

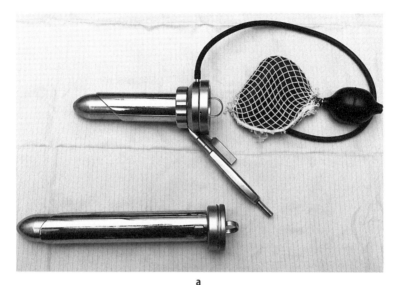

a

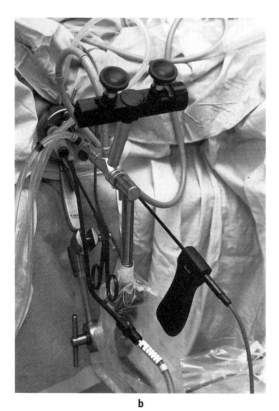

b

Fig. 6.2a,b. Equipment for transanal endoscopic microsurgery. **a** Proctoscopes (12- and 20-cm) shown with obturators; **b** the equipment mounted for use on the Martin arm.

Instruments

The instruments have been specifically designed for endoscopic work. Scissors and forceps are angled to the left or right and the needle holder, forceps and suction device are curved to permit easy access to the pelvic cavity. Silver clips are applied to the thread to avoid the need for surgical knots and a monofilament absorbable suture is used.

Combined Endosurgical Unit

A single unit has been developed that permits pressure-controlled gas dilatation of the rectum. Carbon dioxide can be insufflated at up to 6 litres per minute to maintain rectal pressure between 12 and 15 mmHg. The unit monitors intrarectal pressure and is also connected to a roller pump which provides suction at a lower rate than the insufflation so that suction does not deflate the rectum and obscure the field of view. Standard suction equipment would lead to rapid decompression of the rectum.

Stereoscopic Telescope

One of the major differences between TEM and other minimal access procedure is that the operative field is viewed through a binocular stereoscope. This gives a clear image with the perception of depth of field far superior to that obtained on the video screen during laparoscopic procedures. The image is magnified by up to sixfold. A teaching arm may be attached allowing the assistant to view the operation directly through the optic or via a video screen. Water can be injected automatically through a rinse channel to clean the optics. The optics are angled at approximately 72° so the patient must be placed such that the operative field is positioned inferiorly.

Patient Preparation

Bowel Preparation

Full bowel preparation is needed to prevent faecal contents coming into contact with the mesorectal fat. Buess[27] has advocated the use of 10 litres of normal saline via a nasogastric tube but the more conventional use of a clear fluid diet, laxatives such as sodium picosulphate and enemas is usually sufficient. Colonoscopy should be performed, at the time of admission if possible, to confirm the suitability, level and size of the lesion to be removed. In addition it helps to exclude a synchronous lesion. If the tumour is bulky the top can be removed with a snare at the time of colonoscopy. This will facilitate subsequent TEM without compromising the ability to determine the adequacy of excision since the radial and deep margins of the TEM specimen will not have been affected.

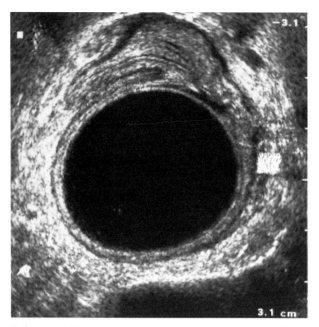

Fig. 6.3. Rectal ultrasound showing a polypoid adenoma (top); there is no evidence of invasion.

Endoluminal Ultrasound

A rectal ultrasound should be performed to assess the lesion for invasion (Fig. 6 3).[28] Overall this is 80–90% accurate at staging the depth of invasion.[29–32] Sailer et al.[33] found an 81% sensitivity and 98% specificity for T1 lesions although there was a tendency to overstage T2 tumours. Peritumoral tissue reaction may be a cause for overstaging,[34,35] and a recent report suggests that with care this area can be distinguished from invasive tumour.[34] Foci of carcinoma within adenomas have been difficult to pick up with a sensitivity of only 50% but a specificity of 94%[36] although sensitivity could be improved with a clear image. Accuracy of endoluminal ultrasound is also greater if the lesion is situated in the upper rectum although the circumferential position of the tumour has been shown to have no effect.[37] However, the examination is not as good at identifying involved lymph nodes, with an accuracy of only 60–80%.[29,30,35,38]

Anaesthesia

Assembly of equipment may be time-consuming and it takes a while to adapt to the TEM instrumentation. In the initial stages therefore, general anaesthesia is preferable to avoid these time constraints. Increasing familiarity with both the equipment and the technique makes it theoretically possible to perform the operation under regional anaesthesia, although the consequent increase in sphincter pressure and ability of the patient to cough may make the procedure even more demanding.

Position of the Patient

The bevel of the sigmoidoscope must face downwards and the position of the patient on the operating table therefore depends upon the location of the tumour in the rectum. For a posterior lesion, the patient is placed in the lithotomy position; for anterior lesions the patient is placed prone with legs apart and the foot of the table dropped to allow the surgeon to sit between the legs; for lesions on the lateral wall the patient is positioned in the lateral position with legs extended on to a side attachment of the table.

Consent

In addition to transanal endoscopic excision of the lesion, consent should be obtained for full laparotomy. If the procedure is technically difficult, there is uncontrollable bleeding or the bowel wall is perforated is may be necessary to perform a laparotomy. That said, some perforations may be repaired with TEM.

Antibiotic Prophylaxis

No studies have been performed to assess the best regime for antibiotic therapy. We use three 8-hourly doses of cefuroxime 750 mg and metronidazole 500 mg starting at the time of operation and then converting to oral co-amoxiclav 500 mg orally for 5 days.

Summary: Preoperative Checklist

- Full bowel preparation
- Colonoscopy at time of admission
- Endoluminal ultrasound
- Full consent
- Antibiotic prophylaxis

Case Selection

Lesions up to 20 cm on the posterior rectal wall may be removed with TEM. However, care must be exercised anteriorly where the upper rectum is intraperitoneal and the risk of free perforation consequently greater (Fig. 6.4).

Adenoma

The large sessile adenoma is the classical indication for TEM. Preoperative assessment with rectal ultrasound is needed to exclude elements of invasion. A partial or full thickness excision may be preferable for larger tumours as early invasion

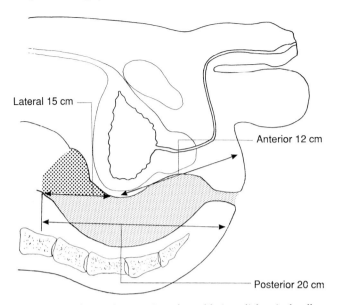

Lateral 15 cm

Anterior 12 cm

Posterior 20 cm

Fig. 6.4. Diagram showing safe area for resection of rectal lesions: light stipple, all tumours; heavy stipple, care should be take anteriorly and laterally beyond 12 cm to avoid intraperitoneal perforation.

may be found in up to 20% of such adenomas.[39] Thicker specimens are also less likely to fragment enabling the pathologist to assess more accurately the margins of resection. Lesions less than 3 cm diameter are the optimum size for removal although it is technically possible to excise much larger tumours. Circumferential lesions can be removed although this will require repositioning of the patient and may predispose to rectal stenosis.

Carcinoma

Four subgroups of patients for local excision of rectal carcinoma have been defined. First, patients with a good chance of curative excision. Essentially this means those patients at low risk of lymph node metastases. To date this has included patients with T1 tumours less than 3 cm in diameter and of good or moderate differentiation with no lymphatic or vascular invasion. Hermanek and Gall[40] found lymph node metastases in only 3% of patients fulfilling these criteria although other reports suggest that 11–12% of T1 tumours have lymph node metastases.[41,42] Kikuchi et al.[43] subdivided T1 carcinomas into three according to the depth of invasion (Fig. 6.5); sm1 is slight submucosal invasion of 200–300 μm, sm2 is intermediate and sm3 has carcinoma invasion near the inner surface of the muscularis propria. Lymph node involvement has not been found in sm1 lesions. The reproducibility of the assessment of these lesions needs to be determined but such a subclassification of T1 lesions may allow more accurate advice on expected outcome of local excision.

The second group consists of patients with a lower chance of curative excision but represent a high risk for major resection or are elderly. Such patients have T2 tumours. The third group are those in whom treatment from the outset is aimed at being palliative only. These patients have large mobile T3 tumours. Finally, there are

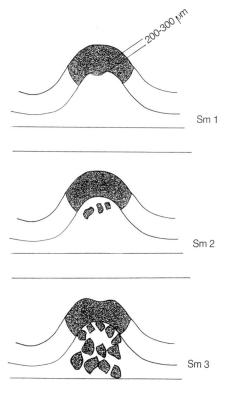

Fig. 6.5. Subclassification of T1 carcinomas (after Kikuchi et al.[43]): sm1, invasion of 200–300 μm; sm2, intermediate; sm3, invasion near the inner surface of the muscularis propria.

a group in whom an incidental carcinoma is discovered following removal of a large adenoma. These are usually T1 tumours and further resection may be unnecessary.

Summary: Cancers Suitable for Potentially Curative Resection by TEM

- T1 lesions
- Less than 3 cm
- Well or moderately differentiated
- No vascular or lymphatic invasion

Technical Considerations

Mucosectomy

Villous lesions may be removed by dissecting in the submucosal plane. A 5-mm margin should be marked out around the circumference of the lesion with the diathermy tip prior to commencing dissection. The mucosa is then elevated using a tissue grasper and the diathermy point used to dissect the lesion in the submucosal plane. For larger villous lesions with an increased risk of occult carcinoma the dissection can be deepened to include part of the muscularis propria. A plane can be developed between the circular and longitudinal muscle layers. Early reports on TEM include data from both mucosectomy and partial thickness excisions. However, we now perform full-thickness excisions in all cases. Care must be taken when dissecting anteriorly not to enter the abdominal cavity, particularly in women, where the peritoneal reflection is low. The posterior vaginal wall is also at risk when dissecting anteriorly in the lower rectum.

Frequent repositioning of the sigmoidoscope is necessary to keep the lesion in the field of view. Irrigation and suction also maintain a good view. Defects may be closed with a continuous 3/0 absorbable suture such as polydiaxone. Short lengths of material should be used in order to maintain tension of the suture in the limited space available. The ends are fixed with a malleable silver clip to avoid the need for knots.

Full-Thickness Resection

Dissection can be extended into the perirectal fat to include lymph nodes from the mesorectum. Although acquisition of lymph nodes was initially popular we have now stopped attempting to obtain nodes so that the mesorectal plane remains undisturbed, thereby allowing unhindered subsequent classical resection should it be deemed necessary. This technique is now our preferred method of excision of all villous tumours and early rectal cancers. The principles of dissection are otherwise the same and particular care must be taken when dissecting anteriorly.

The main intraoperative complications encountered are perforation and haemorrhage. If the peritoneal cavity is breached, it is possible to close the defect endoscopically. In a few cases with a large defect, it may be difficult to maintain adequate distension of the rectum and a laparotomy is then required. Intraoperative bleeding directly obscures the field of view and absorbs light, making subsequent procedures difficult to perform. Most bleeding can be dealt with endoscopically with diathermy haemostasis although it is occasionally necessary to underrun the vessel; a laparotomy is seldom required.

Instrument Handling

It is important to maintain control of the needle at all times and the needle should be passed from instrument to instrument; it is difficult to retrieve and reposition the needle on the needle holder if it is dropped. Crossing of instruments should also be avoided. Cutting and suturing are technically easier when working from right to left. Frequent repositioning of the scope may be necessary. Swapping the instruments round, with the diathermy point through the left port, may facilitate dissection in the left corner.

Training

The technical aspects of the operation are demanding. Unlike other minimal access procedures the instruments are controlled by fine movements of the wrists

and hands rather than from the shoulders and elbows in conventional laparoscopic operations. Whilst there is no substitute for supervised operating in
theatre, Buess has developed a graduated training course as a first line where use
of a training dummy takes participants through a series of graduated exercises
from initial excision of an area from a flat piece of cloth to procedures on intact
animal bowel.[44] Acquisition of the skill from the teaching video screen in theatre
is limited by the non-stereoscopic view and attendance at some form of course is
recommended for anyone contemplating performing TEM. Courses combine the
opportunity of repeated training using the dummy together with instructional
videotapes. With the expanding interest in TEM in the UK, the Royal College of
Surgeons has developed a course run along similar lines which has grown in
popularity since its inception.

Processing of the Specimen

TEM permits complete removal of a specimen enabling the pathologist to assess
completeness of excision both in terms of radial margins and depth of excision.
Once removed, the specimen should be pinned flat on a cork plate (Fig. 6.6) with
the thin rim of normal mucosa pinned in its entirety. The muscularis mucosae
and muscularis propria contract more than the overlying mucosa, which curls up
causing confusion when examining resection margins. Communication between
the pathologist and surgeon can be greatly enhanced if the pathologist is able to
come to theatre to retrieve the specimen. The specimen should be fixed for at least
24 hours before cutting as this greatly improves tissue handling. The deep margin
should be marked, usually with gelatine, and the specimen cut using a long-
bladed sharp knife. The whole specimen should be processed and multiple sections are needed so that the completeness of resection can be determined.

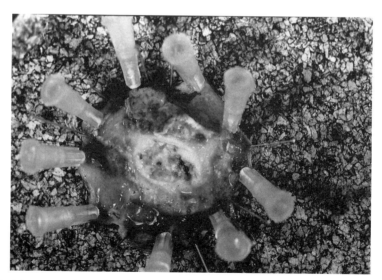

Fig. 6.6. Adenoma specimen pinned out on a cork plate. The top of the lesion had previously been
removed via the colonoscope to reduce the bulk of the lesion.

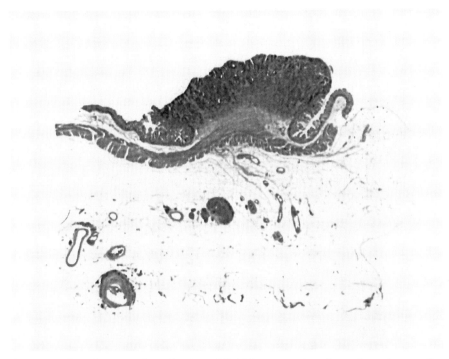

Fig. 6.7. Histological TEM specimen showing a full-thickness resection of an early carcinoma with a lymph node metastasis. The patient subsequently had an anterior resection.

The important objectives of the pathologist are to assess the type of tissue, nature of the lesion, the grade of dysplasia and the presence of invasive elements within the specimen. Lymph nodes are occasionally present in the specimen and their presence and involvement by tumour should be commented upon (Fig. 6.7). Diathermy artefact can occasionally cause confusion[45] but with care the adequacy of excision can be determined with confidence. Similarly, artefact due to trauma from the grasping forceps may give rise to elements of pseudoinvasion or pseudovascular invasion.

Summary: Processing the Specimen

- Immediately pin specimen on cork plate using multiple pins
- Fix for at least 24 hours
- Multiple sections are needed from all areas of the specimen
- Beware of diathery and grasping forceps artefacts

Results

The largest published series on TEM come from Germany[46–50] although other reports are appearing in the literature from the UK[51], USA[52,53] and Italy.[54] It has been technically possible to complete the procedure in the majority of cases. Reports do, however, suggest that initial experience may lead to failure of the procedure in 7–9% of cases[51,53] but rate of conversion to laparotomy is reduced with increased experience with the procedure.[50] The reasons for this include an inadequate seal around the sigmoidoscope because the lesion was too low, large polypoid lesions preventing adequate visualisation and stricturing preventing access, especially in cases of recurrent villous adenoma after previous resection.

Operating Times

The mean operating times depend upon the type of procedure being performed. Average operating time takes around 80 minutes,[26,51] the minimum time 20 minutes and the maximum 240 minutes. Full or partial thickness excisions take longer to perform than mucosal excisions.

Perioperative Complications

The true incidence of free perforation is difficult to determine as many defects are repaired endoscopically and consequently are not reported. The number of procedures requiring conversion to laparotomy is of the order of 1–2%. Bleeding may be encountered in 0–3% of cases but again this can usually be dealt with via the endoscope. Suture disruption has been reported in 0–3% of cases but this can usually be treated conservatively. Occasionally it is necessary to defunction the rectum following suture disruption. Rectovaginal fistulae have been reported in 1–2% of cases and urinary dysfunction requiring catheterisation in up to 4%. Overall complication rates are 7–13% but the number requiring surgery is around 5–6% (Table 6.2). Deaths have been reported in less than 1% of patients but most of these have been cardiopulmonary complications and none have been directly attributable to the procedure itself.[26,49,51,53]

These complication rates are similar to other methods of local excision. The overall complication rate for conventional transanal surgery is 0–14.5% (Table 6.3).[23,39,55-57] The morbidity of anterior resection and APER is far higher and in some series exceeds 50% although the majority of these complications can be treated conservatively.[2,3,58]

Functional Outcome

Transient incontinence occurs in 3–4% of patients undergoing TEM but this usually recovers by one year. Buess and Mentges[26] reported incontinence in 13 of 321 patients undergoing TEM of whom 12 were incontinent to liquid or solids. The incontinence improved in 12 of the 13 patients over the first 5 months. Similarly Steele et al.[51] described initial experience of TEM in the UK with 2 of 100 patients experiencing transient incontinence to flatus.

Manometric studies have shown an initial reduction in both maximum resting and maximum squeeze pressures in the first 48 hours after operation.[59] Despite some evidence suggesting that maximum resting pressure returns to normal by

Table 6.2. Results of transanal endoscopic microsurgery (TEM)

Reference	Year	No. of patients	Proportion of adenomas (%)	Duration of follow-up	Perioperative complications (%)	Incontinence (%)	Mortality (%)	Recurrence of adenoma (%)
Buess and Mentges[26]	1992	317	72	3 months–5 years	6.9	4.1	0.3	5.7
Salm et al.[50]	1994	1900	74	ns	5.7	0.6	0.2	ns
Said and Stippel[49]	1995	260	100	3 months–10 years	6.1	ns	0	6.5
Smith et al.[53]	1996	153	54	ns	8.5	2.0	0	11
Steele et al.[52]	1996	100	77	0–2 years	7	2.0	1	5.2

ns, not stated.

Table 6.3. Results of conventional transanal excision of rectal adenoma

Reference	Year	Technique	No. of patients	Proportion of adenomas (%)	duration of follow-up	Compilcations (%)	Recurrence (%)
Parks and Stuart[39]	1973	Submucosal excision	30	83	6 month–10 years	0	10
Nivatvongs et al.[55]	1973	Submucosal excision	53	94	0–10 years	3.7	9.4
Thomson[23]	1977	Various techniques	106	100	0–10 years	9.5	17.9
Pollard et al.[56]	1988	Various techniques	70	100	0–18 years	ns	13
Sakamoto et al.[57]	1991	Various techniques	117	100	0–15 years	14.4	27.3

ns, not stated.

6 weeks, larger prospective series have shown that resting pressures are diminished 3 and 12 months postoperatively.[60,61] Maximum squeeze pressure was reduced at 3 months but recovered to preoperative values by 12 months.[61] There are no studies using anal ultrasound to compare the sphincters pre- and postoperatively although the manometric studies suggest that there is a degree of damage, particularly to the internal anal sphincter. Although the mean age of patients undergoing TEM is about 65 years, the damage could potentially predispose to incontinence after a longer follow-up.

Functional assessment 3 months postoperatively following anterior resection have shown a significant increase in incontinence to flatus, bowel frequency and use of sanitary pads.[62] Similar results have been reported by Williamson et al.[63] and 29% of their patients had a degree of faecal leakage 1 year after surgery. Direct comparisons of the two procedures is difficult because the anterior resection is usually performed for more advanced disease.

TEM for Adenomas

The majority of reports on TEM describe initial experience with the technique and therefore include data both from adenomas and early rectal cancers. There have been a number of reports from Buess's group, the largest of which describes the results of TEM on 229 adenomas.[26] If the polyps were less than 3 cm a mucosectomy was performed otherwise a full-thickness excision was undertaken except in the intraperitoneal part of the rectum anteriorly where the dissection was restricted to a partial wall excision to avoid entering the peritoneal cavity. Follow-up examinations were performed annually. The majority of tumours were in the mid-rectum although resections were performed up to 24 cm from the anal verge. At follow-up seven (3.1%) recurrent adenomas were seen. A further 13 (5.7%) adenomas were found at new sites in the rectum. Of these adenomas 17 were removed by snare or hot biopsy, two with TEM and one woman had an anterior resection. Said and Stippel[49] described similar recurrence rates following TEM for 260 adenomas. One year actuarial recurrence rate was 1.2% with a 5 year recurrence rate of 7%.

Similar recurrence rates have been reported outside Germany (Table 6.2). Steele et al.[51] found recurrence in 4 of 77 (5.2%) adenomas during a median follow-up of 6 months. Three of these occurred in patients whose operation had been performed for recurrent disease and two had had histologically incomplete excisions. Smith et al.[53] described initial experience of TEM from six centres in the USA. Recurrence rate for adenoma was 11% (9 of 82) of which six were treated by repeat TEM and three by colonoscopic excision. The recurrence rates following TEM for adenoma therefore seem to be between 3 and 11% but increase with length of follow-up. There are three possible mechanisms of recurrence; inadequate excision of the primary lesion, implantation of tumour at the time of the initial TEM, and large adenoma being associated with a mucosal field change thereby increasing the likelihood of further adenomas developing in that area. Many authors do not distinguish between true recurrence at the site of original surgery and a metachronous lesion. Nevertheless, the appearance of further lesions emphasises the need for meticulous follow-up. The main alternative to TEM for local excision of rectal adenomas is Parks's transanal excision of the lesion. As can be seen from Tables 6.2 and 6.3 the recurrence rates for TEM compared favourably with those following conventional transanal surgery. TEM has an additional advantage over traditional techniques in that it also permits resection of lesions from the upper rectum.

TEM for Early Rectal Cancer

Although TEM was initially developed for the removal of large rectal adenomas, in recent years there has been increasing debate on its applicability to the removal of early rectal cancers. At the heart of the debate lies the risk of local recurrence compared with other more traditional methods. Furthermore, although a few mesorectal lymph nodes may be removed with the specimen, total mesorectal excision, which has become the gold standard for rectal cancers, is clearly not possible with TEM. Potentially curative local resections may be undertaken on the basis of risk of lymph node metastases. In T1 tumours lymph node metastases have been found in 3–12% of resected specimens.[40–42]

Mentges et al.[64] have published data from various periods over the past 15 years the most recent of which is summarised in Table 6.4. Nine of 64 T1 carcinomas, 20 of 33 T2 and 9 of 16 T3 tumours underwent further resection. The decision to offer further surgery was based on involvement of resection margins by tumour or at the request of the patient if the postoperative diagnosis of a carcinoma had not been determined preoperatively. Re-resection was not performed in patients with high-risk T1 tumours or higher stages in those of advanced age or with concurrent medical problems. Of the low-risk cancers 2 of 52 T1 tumours, none of 13 T2 and 2 of 4 T3 tumours recurred locally. Patients with recurrence of T1 tumours underwent salvage surgery with curative intent.

Steele et al.[51] reported local recurrence in 2 of 14 T2 carcinomas; both patients had subsequent salvage abdominoperineal excision of the rectum. A further patient with an incomplete excision also underwent abdominoperineal excision of the rectum and was found to have residual tumour in the specimen. Nine of the 14 patients had postoperative radiotherapy as this has been shown to reduce recurrence in following other methods of local excision.[65] There were no cases of local recurrence in the seven patients who had T1 carcinomas removed.

Smith et al.[53] reported higher recurrence rates for all stages of tumours. Ten per cent of T1 tumours, 40% of T2 and 66% of T3 tumours recurred although the numbers were small in the T2 and T3 groups. Those considered good candidates for laparotomy underwent either low anterior resection or abdominoperineal excision.

In a direct comparison of TEM and anterior resection for T1 tumours,[66] local recurrence occurred in one of 24 (4.1%) of TEM patients and distant metastases in one of 26 undergoing anterior resection. Five year survival rates of 96% were similar for both groups but there was a reduced blood loss, operative time, inpatient stay and analgesia requirement in those undergoing TEM.

Graham et al.[67] analysed 10 reports of local excision for rectal cancer. Six per cent of lesions treated were T3 tumours. Methods of excision varied but local recurrence was found in 0–27% of cases. Absolute survival rates ranged from 65 to 100% but cancer-specific survival was 82–100%. Positive margins in the surgical specimen, poorly differentiated histology and increased depth of invasion were associated with a significant increase in mortality and local recurrence. The figures for local recurrence and mortality following TEM compare favourably with other methods of local excision.

Table 6.4. Results of reoperation after local treatment for 113 rectal carcinomas and subsequent follow-up of those patients undergoing local excision of carcinomas

Tumour stage	Number	Re-operated	Residual primary tumour	Lymph node metastases	No. followed up after local excision only	Local recurrence
T1 Low-risk	60	8	2	0	52	2
T1 High-Risk	4	1	0	0	3	0
T2 Low-risk	31	18	2	5	13	0
T2 High-risk	2	2	0	0	0	0
T3 Low-risk	13	9	1	2	4	2
T3 High-risk	3	1	0	0	2	0
Total	113	39				

From Mentges et al.[64]

Alternative forms of local therapy for rectal cancer have been employed. Papillon[68] described his initial experience with endocavitary radiation in 1973 with a five year survival of 72% and local recurrence in 7%. Subsequent reports from Papillon[69] and Sischy et al.[70,71] have confirmed these results in low risk patients. However, endocavitary irradiation does not provide a complete specimen; histology is limited to random biopsies and depth of invasion determined by endoluminal ultrasound. Since accurate pathological staging is not possible it is difficult to compare this mode of treatment directly with TEM.

Comparison must also be made with low anterior resection and total mesorectal excision for which a selected personal series reports 5-year local recurrence rates of 4%[72] but a higher morbidity. TEM can be offered to a selected group of patients with low-risk T1 tumours with a similar low local recurrence rates and 5-year survival of over 90%. The role of TEM in potentially curative procedures for high-risk T1 and T2 tumours has yet to be clarified although radiotherapy may improve the results in these lesions.[65,73] Willett et al.[74] found similar survival for low-risk T1 and T2 tumours treated by local excision compared with treatment by APER. However, for high-risk lesions (poorly differentiated, vascular or lymphatic invasion) APER had a superior outcome. Nevertheless, the low recurrence rates and 5-year survival of more than 90% serve to justify local resection in T1 tumours.

TEM for Palliation of Rectal Carcinoma

TEM has been used as a means of palliation for more advanced rectal cancers.[75] The theoretical advantages are that it offers palliation for large tumour without the need for major surgery. Transanal resection of tumours using an adapted urological resectoscope resulted in a similar 5-year survival when compared APER in an elderly population.[76,77] Although repeated resections may be needed, the procedure may be performed quickly and with minimal morbidity. By definition, excision of the lesion is incomplete and consequently piecemeal excision is acceptable. At present there is no evidence that TEM has an advantage over this other form of minimal access surgery for palliative procedures.

Postoperative Stay and Follow-up

In-patient stay following TEM depends upon the procedure performed. Patients require a longer hospital stay and more gradual introduction of oral feeding following a full-thickness excision than after mucosectomy. In-patient stay following TEM is a median of 2–4 days.[51,53]

Follow-up of patients after TEM is mandatory because of the potential for recurrent disease. Many of the recurrent adenomas seen at follow-up are small and can be treated by snare polypectomy. The site of TEM can be visualised through the rigid sigmoidoscope in out-patients and we would advocate a 6 week and 6 month out-patient appointment with follow-up colonoscopy at 12 months. A similar protocol can be used for completely excised T1 carcinomas.

Management of Recurrent Disease

There is no theoretical limit to number of times TEM can be used for recurrent lesions but the risk of stenosis may increase with repeated surgery. Data on recurrent disease are sparse, but if a large adenoma recurred more than twice it may be prudent to proceed to anterior resection as a definitive treatment.

Patients with low-risk T1 carcinomas who undergo re-resection have a worse local recurrence rate of more than 10%. Local recurrence of carcinoma should probably be dealt with by salvage anterior resection or APER. This is potentially curable in over 50% of patients.[78] However, if unfavourable features are present in the original local resection specimen, early intervention has a better outcome than subsequent salvage surgery.[78]

Conclusions

TEM has extended the boundaries of minimal access surgery in the rectum. It permits the complete removal of large sessile adenomas in patients who may previously have undergone anterior resection or APER. Coupled with this are low complication rates and low incidence of local recurrence compared with other forms of local excision. Its use can also be justified in the treatment of low-risk T1 tumours but as yet there is insufficient evidence for it to be used as a curative procedure for high-risk T1 and T2 lesions. Further assessment of these lesions should be performed within properly constructed trials. The equipment is expensive to purchase and the technique takes time to master. Consequently, for the time being it should remain a treatment option in only a few centres, each of which perform sufficient numbers of procedures per year to maintain a good outcome.

References

1. Buess G, Hutterer F, Theiss J, Bobel M, Isselhard W, Pichlmaier H (1984) A system for a transanal endoscopic rectum operation. Chirurg 55:677–680.
2. Gillen P, Peel AL (1986) Comparison of the mortality, morbidity and incidence of local recurrence in patients with rectal cancer treated by either stapled anterior resection or abdominoperineal resection. Br J Surg 73:339–341.
3. Hughes ES, McDermott FT, Masterton JP, Cunningham IG, Polglase AL (1980) Operative mortality following excision of the rectum. Br J Surg 67:49–51.
4. Lea JWT, Covington K, McSwain B, Scott HW Jr (1982) Surgical experience with carcinoma of the colon and rectum. Ann Surg 195:600–607.
5. Ohman U (1982) Colorectal carcinoma – trends and results over a 30-year period. Dis Colon Rectum 25:431–440.
6. Payne JE, Chapuis PH, Pheils MT (1986) Surgery for large bowel cancer in people aged 75 years and older. Dis Colon Rectum 29:733–737.
7. Yeager ES, Van Heerden JA (1980) Sexual dysfunction following proctocolectomy and abdominoperineal resection. Ann Surg 191:169–170.
8. Kinn AC, Ohman U (1986) Bladder and sexual function after surgery for rectal cancer. Dis Colon Rectum 29:43–48.
9. Marks CG, Ritchie JK (1975) The complications of synchronous combined excision for adenocarcinoma of the rectum at St Mark's Hospital. Br J Surg 62:901–905.
10. Kraske P (1885) Zur Extirpation hochsitzender Mastdarmkrebse. Verh Dtsch Ges Chir 14:464–474.

11. Christiansen J (1980) Excision of mid-rectal lesions by the Kraske sacral approach. Br J Surg 67:651–652.
12. Westbrook KC, Lang NP, Broadwater JR, Thompson BW (1982) Posterior surgical approaches to the rectum. Ann Surg 195:677–685.
13. Mason AY (1970) Surgical access to the rectum – a transsphincteric exposure. Proc R Soc Med 63:91–94.
14. Geenen JE, Schmitt MG, Jr., Wu WC, Hogan WJ (1975) Major complications of colonoscopy: bleeding and perforation. Am J Dig Dis 20:231–235.
15. Nivatvongs S (1988) Complications in colonoscopic polypectomy: lessons to learn from an experience with 1576 polyps. Am Surg 54:61–63.
16. Shirai M, Nakamura T, Matsuura A, Ito Y, Kobayashi S (1994) Safer colonoscopic polypectomy with local submucosal injection of hypertonic saline-epinephrine solution. Am J Gastroenterol 89:334–338.
17. Binmoeller KF, Bohnacker S, Seifert H, Thonke F, Valdeyar H, Soehendra N (1996) Endoscopic snare excision of "giant" colorectal polyps. Gastrointest Endosc 43:183–188.
18. Irwin RJ (1984) Resectoscopic transanal resection of extensive rectal adenomas. Aust N Z J Surg 54:375–377.
19. Stephenson BM, Ng KJ, Shandall AA, Price Thomas JM (1992) Endoscopic transanal resection of large villous tumours of the rectum. Ann R Coll Surg Engl 74:54–58.
20. Brunetaud JM, Maunoury V, Cochelard D, Boniface B, Cortot A, Paris JC (1989) Endoscopic laser treatment for rectosigmoid villous adenoma: factors affecting the results. Gastroenterology 97:272–277.
21. Brunetaud JM, Maunoury V, Cochelard D (1995) Lasers in rectosigmoid tumors. Semin Surg Oncol 11:319–327.
22. Keck JO, Schoetz DJ Jr, Roberts PL, Murray JJ, Coller JA, Veidenheimer MC (1995) Rectal mucosectomy in the treatment of giant rectal villous tumors. Dis Colon Rectum 38:233–238.
23. Thomson JP (1977) Treatment of sessile villous and tubulovillous adenomas of the rectum: experience of St. Mark's Hospital. 1963–1972. Dis Colon Rectum 20:467–472.
24. Parks AG (1968) A technique for excising extensive villous papillomatous change in the lower rectum. Proc R Soc Med 61:441–442.
25. Buess G, Kipfmuller K, Hack D, Grussner R, Heintz A, Junginger T (1988) Technique of transanal endoscopic microsurgery. Surg Endosc 2:71–75.
26. Buess GF, Mentges B (1992) Transanal endoscopic microsurgery (TEM). Minimally Invasive Therapy 1:101–109.
27. Buess G (1993) Review: transanal endoscopic microsurgery (TEM). JR Coll Surg Edinb 38:239–245.
28. Beynon J, Foy DM, Roe AM, Temple LN, Mortensen NJ (1986) Endoluminal ultrasound in the assessment of local invasion in rectal cancer. Br J Surg 73:474–477.
29. Holdsworth PJ, Johnston D, Chalmers AG, Chennells P, Dixon MF, Finan PJ, et al. (1988) Endoluminal ultrasound and computed tomography in the staging of rectal cancer. Br J Surg 75:1019–1022.
30. Thaler W, Watzka S, Martin F et al. (1994) Preoperative staging of rectal cancer by endoluminal ultrasound vs. magnetic resonance imaging. Preliminary results of a prospective, comparative study. Dis Colon Rectum 37:1189–1193.
31. Starck M, Bohe M, Fork FT, Lindstrom C, Sjoberg S (1995) Endoluminal ultrasound and low-field magnetic resonance imaging are superior to clinical examination in the preoperative staging of rectal cancer. Eur J Surg 161:841–845.
32. Solomon MJ, McLeod RS (1993) Endoluminal transrectal ultrasonography: accuracy, reliability, and validity. Dis Colon Rectum 36:200–205.
33. Sailer M, Leppert R, Kraemer M, Fuchs KH, Thiede A (1997) The value of endorectal ultrasound in the assessment of adenomas, T1- and T2-carcinomas. Int J Colorectal Dis 12:214–219.
34. Maier AG, Barton PP, Neuhold NR, Herbst F, Teleky BK, Lechner GL (1997) Peritumoral tissue reaction at transrectal US as a possible cause of overstaging in rectal cancer: histopathologic correlation. Radiology 203:785–789.
35. Akasu T, Sugihara K, Moriya Y, Fujita S (1997) Limitations and pitfalls of transrectal ultrasonography for staging of rectal cancer. Dis Colon Rectum 40:S10–S15.
36. Adams WJ, Wong WD (1995) Endorectal ultrasonic detection of malignancy within rectal villous lesions. Dis Colon Rectum 38:1093–1096.
37. Sailer M, Leppert R, Bussen D, Fuchs KH, Thiede A (1997) Influence of tumor position on accuracy of endorectal ultrasound staging. Dis Colon Rectum 40:1180–1186.
38. Herzog U, von Flue M, Tondelli P, Schuppisser JP (1993) How accurate is endorectal ultrasound in the preoperative staging of rectal cancer? Dis Colon Rectum 36:127–134.

39. Parks AG, Stuart AE (1973) The management of villous tumours of the large bowel. Br J Surg 60:688–695.
40. Hermanek P, Gall FP (1986) Early (microinvasive) colorectal carcinoma. Pathology, diagnosis, surgical treatment. Int J Colorectal Dis 1:79–84.
41. Brodsky JT, Richard GK, Cohen AM, Minsky BD (1992) Variables correlated with the risk of lymph node metastasis in early rectal cancer. Cancer 69:322–326.
42. Huddy SP, Husband EM, Cook MG, Gibbs NM, Marks CG, Heald RJ (1993) Lymph node metastases in early rectal cancer. Br J Surg 80:1457–1458.
43. Kikuchi R, Takano M, Koichi T et al. (1995) Management of early invasive colorectal cancer. Dis Colon Rectum 38:1286–1295.
44. Kipfmuller K, Buess G, Naruhn M, Junginger T (1988) Training program for transanal endoscopic microsurgery. Surg Endosc 2:24–27.
45. Burd E, Warren BF, Mountford RA, Durdey P, Bradfield JW, Sheppard NA (1990) Hot biopsy forceps artifact in the colon – a cause of diagnostic confusion. J Pathol 167:110A.
46. Buess G, Kipfmuller K, Ibald R et al. (1988) Clinical results of transanal endoscopic microsurgery. Surg Endosc 2:245–250.
47. Buess G, Mentges B, Manncke K, Starlinger M, Becker HD (1992) Technique and results of transanal endoscopic microsurgery in early rectal cancer. Am J Surg 163:63–70.
48. Said S, Huber P, Pichlmaier H (1993) Technique and clinical results of endorectal surgery. Surgery 113:65–75.
49. Said S, Stippel D (1995) Transanal endoscopic microsurgery in large, sessile adenomas of the rectum. A 10-year experience. Surg Endosc 9:1106–1112.
50. Salm R, Lampe H, Bustos A, Matern U (1994) Experience with TEM in Germany. Endosc Surg Allied Technol 2:251–254.
51. Steele RJ, Hershman MJ, Mortensen NJ, Armitage NC, Scholefield JH (1996) Transanal endoscopic microsurgery – initial experience from three centres in the United Kingdom. Br J Surg 83:207–210.
52. Saclarides TJ, Smith L, Ko ST, Orkin B, Buess G (1992) Transanal endoscopic microsurgery. Dis Colon Rectum 35:1183–1191.
53. Smith LE, Ko ST, Saclarides T, Caushaj P, Orkin BA, Khanduja KS (1996) Transanal endoscopic microsurgery. Initial registry results. Dis Colon Rectum 39:S79–S84.
54. Chiavellati L, D'Elia G, Zerilli M, Tremiterra S, Stipa S (1994) Management of large malignant rectal polyps with transanal endoscopic microsurgery. Is there anything better for the patient? Eur J Surg Oncol 20:658–666.
55. Nivatvongs S, Balcos EG, Schottler JL, Goldberg SM (1973) Surgical management of large villous tumors of the rectum. Dis Colon Rectum 16:508–514.
56. Pollard SG, Macfarlane R, Everett WG (1988) Villous tumours of the large bowel. Br J Surg 75:910–912.
57. Sakamoto GD, MacKeigan JM, Senagore AJ (1991) Transanal excision of large, rectal villous adenomas. Dis Colon Rectum 34:880–885.
58. Bokey EL, Chapuis PH, Fung C et al. (1995) Postoperative morbidity and mortality following resection of the colon and rectum for cancer. Dis Colon Rectum 38:480–487.
59. Hemingway D, Flett M, McKee RF, Finlay IG (1996) Sphincter function after transanal endoscopic microsurgical excision of rectal tumours. Br J Surg 83:51–52.
60. Banerjee AK, Jehle EC, Kreis ME et al. (1996) Prospective study of the proctographic and functional consequences of transanal endoscopic microsurgery. Br J Surg 83:211–213.
61. Kreis ME, Jehle EC, Haug V et al. (1996) Functional results after transanal endoscopic microsurgery. Dis Colon Rectum 39:1116–1121.
62. Jehle EC, Haenhel T, Starlinger J, Becker HD (1995) Level of the anastomosis does not influence functional outcome after anterior resection for rectal cancer. Am J Surg 169:147–153.
63. Williamson ME, Lewis WG, Finan PJ, Miller AS, Holdsworth PJ, Johnston D (1995) Recovery of physiologic and clinical function after low anterior resection of the rectum for carcinoma: myth of reality? Dis Colon Rectum 38:411–418.
64. Mentges B, Buess G, Effinger G, Manncke K, Becker HD (1997) Indications and results of local treatment of rectal cancer. Br J Surg 84:348–351.
65. Rouanet P, Saint Aubert B, Fabre JM et al. (1993) Conservative treatment for low rectal carcinoma by local excision with or without radiotherapy. Br J Surg 80:1452–1456.
66. Winde G, Nottberg H, Keller R, Schmid KW, Bunte H (1996) Surgical cure for early rectal carcinomas (T1). Transanal endoscopic microsurgery vs. anterior resection. Dis Colon Rectum 39:969–976.

67. Graham RA, Garnsey L, Jessup JM (1990) Local excision of rectal carcinoma. Am J Surg 160:306–312.
68. Papillon J (1973) Endocavity irradiation of early rectal cancers for cure: a series of 123 cases. Proc R Soc Med 66:1179–1181.
69. Papillon J (1984) New prospects in the conservative treatment of rectal cancer. Dis Colon Rectum 27:695–700.
70. Sischy B, Remington JH, Sobel SH (1978) Treatment of rectal carcinomas by means of endocavity irradiation. Cancer 42:1073–1076.
71. Sischy B, Remington JH, Sobel SH (1980) Treatment of rectal carcinomas by means of endocavitary irradiation: a progress report. Cancer 46:1957–1961.
72. MacFarlane JK, Ryall RD, Heald RJ (1993) Mesorectal excision for rectal cancer. Lancet 341:457–460.
73. Bleday R, Breen E, Jessup JM, Burgess A, Sentovich SM, Steele G (1997) Prospective evaluation of local excision for small rectal cancers. Dis Colon Rectum 40:388–392.
74. Willett CG, Compton CC, Shellito PC, Efird JT (1994) Selection factors for local excision or abdominoperineal resection of early stage rectal cancer. Cancer 73:2716–2720.
75. Turler A, Schafer H, Pichlmaier H (1997) Role of transanal endoscopic microsurgery in the palliative treatment of rectal cancer. Scand J Gastroenterol 32:58–61.
76. Dickinson AJ, Savage AP, Mortensen NJ, Kettlewell MG (1993) Long-term survival after endoscopic transanal resection of rectal tumours. Br J Surg 80:1401–1404.
77. Savage AP, Reece Smith H, Faber RG (1994) Survival after peranal and abdominoperineal resection for rectal carcinoma. Br J Surg 81:1482–1484.
78. Baron PL, Enker WE, Zakowski MF, Urmacher C (1995) Immediate vs. salvage resection after local treatment for early rectal cancer. Dis Colon Rectum 38:177–181.

7 Incontinence Surgery

G.A. Santoro and D.C.C. Bartolo

Introduction

The surgical treatment of incontinence remains somewhat empirical although considerable advances have been made in understanding the pathophysiology of the condition in recent years.[1] The purpose of this chapter is to characterise this disorder and to put into perspective the numerous procedures that have been described for the treatment of this condition.

Anal Incontinence

Anal incontinence is the inability to control the release of bowel contents and it can be partial (liquid and gas) or complete (solid). It is important to differentiate between minor levels of functional loss and the clinical state in which there is a serious disruption of normal life. These may represent different ends of the same spectrum or, alternatively, may be indicative of differing underlying pathologies. Minor degrees of anal incontinence are relatively common especially with increasing age and most patients with minor continence problems can be satisfactorily managed by dietary advice and medication to modify stool consistency. In this section, minor incontinence is defined as the occasional faecal staining of underwear (faecal leakage or soiling or seepage), incontinence of flatus, incontinence in the presence of loose stool only or rectal urgency. Major incontinence is defined as the frequent and inadvertent voiding per anum of formed stool and represents the most severe form of faecal incontinence, for which an active therapeutic approach is advocated.

There are many and varied causes of incontinence.[1] It may be important to categorise the aetiology of incontinence so that an appropriate sphincter repair can be selected. Most patients have acquired anal incontinence, secondary to obstetric laceration, previous anorectal surgery (such as fistulotomy or haemorrhoidectomy) or trauma (such as impalement). These injuries are the most amenable to surgical management, specifically, the anal sphincteroplasty. Other causes of incontinence, such as long-standing prolapse or third to fourth degree haemorrhoids, often respond to treatment of the primary disorder alone. More difficult to treat are neurogenic injuries, such as those resulting from massive neuromuscular trauma, myelomeningocele or demyelinating diseases of the spinal cord, massive infection or vascular accident. The gracilis muscle transposition is the best procedure suited to injuries of this type.

In patients in whom there is no functioning sphincter muscle at all, and in whom it is impractical to create a neosphincter, a defunctioning stoma is often the best option. The latter, of course, is always available to those patients in whom the procedures mentioned before either fail or are contraindicated. Inflammatory conditions, such as chronic ulcerative colitis, Crohn's colitis and amoebic colitis can cause incontinence by the diarrhoea associated with these conditions or because of the decreased compliance of the rectum secondary to inflammation or scarring. Treatment should be aimed at the primary problem, since sphincter repairs are usually neither indicated nor successful. Very difficult to manage is the group of patients presenting with functional incontinence which is mostly idiopathic. These patients exhibit lower resting anal pressures, frequent episodes of transient internal sphincter relaxation combined with electromechanical dissociation of the internal anal sphincter.[2,3]

Diagnosing the cause and assessing the severity of the condition precede any treatment.[4,5] In the history, severity of incontinence should be evaluated. Milder forms of incontinence may respond adequately to non-operative therapy (diet, drugs, bowel training, sphincter exercises, improved hygiene). Digital examination is very important to check for the length, tone and anatomical integrity of anal canal, reaction of puborectalis to straining and coughing, sensibility of anal wall to pressure, presence of faecal loading, evidence of intussusception or prolapse of rectal wall and status of the rectovaginal septum and perineal body in women. Proctoscopy, barium enemas and proctography should be used to rule out tumours, colitis, mucosal rectal prolapse, solitary ulcer syndrome, haemorrhoids or faecal impaction.[6] Assessment of complex sphincter defects can be difficult. Adjunctive investigation such as endoluminal ultrasound (EUS) and needle electromyography (EMG) may provide evidence of the nature and extent of the sphincter defects.[7,8] EUS seems preferable to EMG in mapping these defects and can be a useful adjunct to physiological studies of anorectal function (anal manometry, pudendal nerve terminal motor latency, mucosal electrosensitivity) in patients with faecal incontinence. All these techniques help the clinician in determining whether the incontinence is related to a sphincter deficit, a neurological problem or a combination of both.

When the aetiology and nature of the injury are clear and the incontinence is severe enough, then the appropriate anal sphincter reconstruction operation may be performed.

Surgical Management

Not all patients referred for surgery are candidates for operation. It is therefore the duty of the surgeon to ensure that the patient has received a reasonable trial of medical treatment and that the symptoms are severe enough to warrant operation.[9] There now follows a critical appraisal of the different procedures which are available for the surgical treatment of incontinence.

Anal Sphincteroplasty

The majority of patients who come to sphincter repair present at a late stage to the specialist surgeon. The commonest lesion is anterior division of the external anal sphincter as a result of an obstetric injury by disruption at traumatic delivery, tearing or by misplaced episiotomy.[10] If not recognised and properly repaired the wound will heal by secondary intention and this will result in a deficient anal canal with poor function. Subsequent childbirth may further stretch the pelvic floor and puborectalis muscle and the patient may then present with major faecal incontinence. Development of faecal incontinence may be delayed in other cases until middle age when the pelvic floor muscles naturally begin to deteriorate. Obstetric injury does not usually affect the puborectalis and therefore the incontinence is not as severe as that caused by injury to the lateral and posterior aspects of the sphincter mechanism, as a result of trauma or surgical treatment, which frequently involve the puborectalis muscle.[11]

After traumatic rupture the divided anal sphincter retracts to about half its normal circumference, the gap being bridged by dense fibrous tissue. Preoperative sphincter mapping either by EMG or by EUS may be advantageous if the injury is complex. Historically delayed repair of anal sphincter injury has involved excision of the scar with direct apposition of the muscle ends, but results were disappointing because sutures pulled out of the muscle.[11] Alternative methods were later reported by Blaisdell[12] where scar tissue was not touched, but the sphincter muscle ring was tightened by plication. In 1971 Parks and McPartlin[13] reported much better results with a technique of scar tissue excision, creation of a new anal mucosal tube and an overlapping muscle repair. A routine defunctioning colostomy was used with these patients. Slade et al.[14] and Fang et al.[15] have reported equally good results with a modified overlapping technique without colostomy.

The operation is performed under a general anaesthetic with the patient catheterised and either in the lithotomy or prone jack-knife position.[9] A wide incision centred on the scar tissue is made to encompass about half of the circumference of the anal canal. Dissection is then performed, ensuring that the sphincter has been exposed adequately in its depth as well as in its circumference. The scar tissue is divided vertically down in its length in such a way to recreate the two cut ends of the external sphincter. It is never practicable to try to separate the internal and external sphincters from each other and repair them separately. They should be displayed and repaired as one muscle. The sphincter muscle on each side of the injury must be dissected back for a short distance; great judgement is required to mobilise enough sphincter, but to preserve some fibrous tissue to hold sutures for subsequent repair and to avoid ischaemia of the ends. Excessive mobilisation will render the muscle ischaemic or cause denervation. The epithelial layer is repaired with a continuous run of absorbable sutures. The ends of the mobilised sphincter are united by an overlap technique. Starting at the deepest part of the repair, it is usual to place four sutures in a row about 1 cm apart. Non-absorbable materials such as 2/0 Prolene are suitable. It is probably simplest, however, to perform the repair with materials which absorb over a long period of time such as polydioxanone (PDS). Sometimes it is difficult to judge the degree of overlap. It is better to obtain a good union rather than risk trying to produce an overlap with undue tension. The resulting repair may narrow the canal to approximately half its normal circumference. It is better, indeed, to have a tight anal canal that can always be dilated later, than a repair that is too loose.

Surgeons[1] are now agreed that a colostomy is unnecessary in straightforward cases but should be used in cases of severe perineal trauma and in some highly selected cases of Crohn's disease.

In a series of 97 cases reported by Browning and Motson,[16] 36 patients with traumatic or obstetric injury were treated by a direct overlapping sphincter repair. Of these, 92% were restored to full continence for solid and liquid stool, although some remained incontinent of flatus. In 44 patients followed up after repair for operative injury the results were less good, 66% being continent of solid and liquid stool. Similarly, Keighley and Fielding[17] obtained an 80% overall success rate for this procedure and Henry et al.[1] confirmed the difference in results between the two types of injury. In a retrospective review[18] of 44 patients undergoing overlapping sphincter repair at the Cleveland Clinic a satisfactory continence was attained in 86% of cases. This is comparable with the excellent results reported by Fang et al.[15] at the University of Minnesota in 79 patients treated by this technique. Our own results[19] with 14 traumatic sphincter injuries and 16 cases of idiopathic incontinence demonstrated a satisfactory clinical result in 71% of patients in the traumatic group and in 62% of patients in the idiopathic group. This was associated with a significant increase ($P<0.005$) in maximum voluntary contraction pressure in the traumatic group and in those patients who had a good result in the idiopathic group. Sitzler and Thomson[20] in a recent review of 31 overlap sphincter repairs performed at St Mark's Hospital, achieved a successful outcome in 74% of patients. In their series, postoperative anal manometry was not discriminatory between successful and failed groups. EUS appeared accurate in documenting residual anal sphincter defects in the poor outcome group. Use of a stoma in covering the anal wound while it healed was associated with less infection of the wound, but there was no statistical difference in success rate between those covered by stoma and those not covered.

Associated pudendal nerve injury is the most likely cause for treatment failure in patients undergoing repair of obstetric injuries to the anal sphincter. Sangwan et al.[21] suggested, in a recent report, that both pudendal nerves must be intact to achieve normal continence after sphincter repair. They observed that patients with unilateral pudendal neuropathy are more likely to have poor rather than good postoperative function. Wexner et al.[22] also observed in their series that patients with unilateral prolongation of pudendal nerve terminal motor latency had an unsatisfactory outcome.

For more severe injuries in which the entire sphincter mechanism has been disrupted, a plication of the anterior levator muscles is performed before the overlapping sphincteroplasty. The purpose of adding this levatorplasty in such injury is both to strengthen and lengthen the anal canal, improving continence. Osterberg et al.[23] recently reported long-term results of anterior levatorplasty without overlapping sphincteroplasty in 54 patients with obstetric trauma and 31 patients with idiopathic incontinence. The operative technique consisted of approximating both limbs of the puborectalis and pubococcygeus muscles with two layers of sutures. A good result was achieved in 74% of patients with an obstetric injury and in 45% of patients in the idiopathic group.

Post-anal Repair

It has been suggested that the acute anorectal angle produced by the action of the puborectalis muscle is fundamental to the maintenance of continence by creating a flap-valve effect. According to Parks,[24] idiopathic faecal incontinence was associated with perineal descent and an obtuse anorectal angle which rendered the flap valvular mechanism ineffective. To correct this in 1975 he described the operation of post-anal repair to recreate the acute anorectal angle by plication of the puborectalis and external anal sphincter.

The anatomical key to this operation is the avascular intersphincteric space which separates the internal sphincter from the external sphincter. The dissection can be started and developed in the early stages most easily in the laterally. At the tip of the external sphincter the puborectalis muscle will be identified. As the surgeon enters the supralevator plane, the fascia of Waldayer is seen. This is incised to allow the post-rectal space to be opened up. Once the muscle has been completely exposed, suturing begins with interrupted polypropylene. The first layer approximates the ileococcygeus muscle, the second layer approximates the pubococcygeus muscle and the third layer approximates the puborectalis muscle. It is important that the knot should not be tied too tightly as this will cause necrosis of tissue. A small gap may be left between the approximated muscles so that this will not cause tissue necrosis. Finally the external sphincter is approximated.

Some patients with idiopathic faecal incontinence, however, do not have an obtuse anorectal angle. Furthermore it has been demonstrated by proctographic techniques that the anterior rectal wall is not in contact with the upper anal canal during periods of high intra-abdominal pressure.[25] These findings have led us to conclude that continence is maintained by sphincteric action rather than a flap-valve effect.[26] In studies[27,28] in which we measured the anorectal angle before and after sphincter repair for incontinence, resting and squeeze pressures rose significantly in those with a successful outcome, while the anorectal angle did not alter significantly following successful surgery. Similar success rates were obtained using post-anal repair or anterior sphincteroplasy and levatorplasty. It appeared, therefore, that the obtuse anorectal angle in incontinence was an epiphenomenon representing weakness of the puborectalis. Accordingly, we have modified our approach to the management of incontinence. In the past we have subdivided patients on the basis of clinical, physiological and electromyographic findings into two groups: those with traumatic sphincter disruption and those with idiopathic faecal incontinence. The former were offered anterior sphincter plication and the latter post-anal repair. From 1987 onwards we have used an anterior approach to treat all patients with incontinence, irrespective of the aetiology. Our experience[28] on 17 patients with idiopathic faecal incontinence treated by post-anal repairs demonstrated that resting and squeeze anal canal pressures were improved following post-anal repairs, as was upper sensation, but there was no change in the anorectal angle. Repair was successful in 59% of patients and this is similar to results reported by Browning and Parks[29] in 140 patients who had had a post-anal repair, with 74% of patients continent for solid and liquid stool, 12% of patients incontinent for liquid stool and 14% of patients totally incontinent. Yoshioka and Keighley[30] analysed 61 patients with idiopathic faecal incontinence treated by post-anal repair. A significant improvement was achieved in 90% of patients; however, 57% had urgency, 76% had episodes of leakage, 38%

wore a pad and 62% were unable to discriminate what was passing through the anal canal. They found no correlation between the clinical result and anal canal pressures. They concluded that the quality of continence after post-anal repair is poor. Womack et al.[31] confirmed that the anorectal angle was not consistently found to change significantly after post-anal repair. The only factor which appeared to correlate with improved function was anal canal length. Satisfactory results were reported in 87% of their patients. Rainey et al.[32] published results of 40 patients treated. They suggested that it is probably only in patients with incontinence for solid stool that this operation should be considered, that it would not be of value in those with incontinence for liquid stool and that it would be certainly not be expected to help those with problems of flatus control. Furthermore, these authors showed that functional outcome deteriorated with time in 21% of patients. Yoshioka et al.[33] have demonstrated that after 3 years only 30% of patients still have a successful result. Experience with post-anal repair has been limited at the Cleveland Clinic and the results are poor when compared with those previously reported.[18] Of the nine post-anal repair operations four were complete failures.

Gracilis Muscle Transposition

Traditional therapies are not always efficacious for patients with chronic end-stage faecal incontinence caused by pudendal neuropathy, sphincter trauma or congenital anomalies. For these patients graciloplasty should be considered if standard medical and surgical treatments have failed and gracilis muscle is viable for transposition.[34] This technique was initially described by Pickrell[35] in 1959 who reported success in 50 children and 40 adults. It is possible to use either one (single-sling technique) or both muscles (double-sling technique).

The gracilis muscle is the most superficial muscle on the medial aspect of the thigh. The muscle originates at the pubic tubercle, and its tendon inserts onto the tibia just below the medial condyle and behind the sartorius muscle. Transposition is possible because its neural and vascular supplies enter the proximal portion of the muscle. The neurovascular bundle marks the proximal extent of mobilization. The muscle is brought through a subcutaneous tunnel created between the proximal thigh and the anterior anal incision, wrapped around the external sphincter muscle and attached to the opposite ischial tuberosity. If both muscles are used a strong, wide posterior band of muscular support is provided to the back and sides of the anal tube. If a single muscle of short length is used, it is better to wrap it fully around the anal canal to provide circumferential support and to re-fasten the muscle to itself by overlapping sutures. The anus must be tight enough to admit only one finger. If the anal orifice is too tight it can easily be corrected by dilatation, but if the opening is too lax, incontinence and operative failure will result. Unless the tunnels are wide enough to allow for easy passage of the gracilis slings, the muscle may be damaged by excessive traction at the time of operation. A defaecatory pattern training is necessary to allow patients to evacuate completely and spontaneously. Traditional graciloplasty, however, requires the patient to consciously and continuously contract the transposed gracilis muscle to maintain continence. Further, the muscle may become easily fatigued, resulting in loss of continence.

The results of this operation have been variable. Leguit et al.[36] reported on 10 patients with a 6-month to 17-year follow-up. Ninety per cent of patients were continent to formed faeces, whereas one patient was worsened after the procedure. Good results were also reported by Corman[37] in young patients who had sustained severe perineal trauma necessitating an urgent colostomy (8 out of 14 patients had good or excellent results), but results were far less satisfactory in patients with idiopathic faecal incontinence. Faucheron et al.[38] reviewed 22 patients who underwent gracilis transposition. At 6 months, 18 patients had improved continence, but 12 of 18 were stable with time, and only one was fully continent. Yoshioka and Keighley[39] reported six cases treated with a gracilis muscle transplant with poor functional results in all patients, all of whom were ultimately treated with colostomy. They found no objective improvement in resting or voluntary pressure postoperatively in their patients.

Recently, in an attempt to achieve sustained muscle contraction, implanted portable nerve stimulators have been developed with encouraging early results. Dynamic graciloplasty combines the historical technique of graciloplasty with modern electrical muscle stimulation technology. After a period of muscle conditioning, this new technique produces muscle tissue that is more fatigue-resistant, providing a neo-sphincter that does not require conscious control. An unconditioned skeletal muscle, such as the gracilis, will fatigue under constant contraction. But within a few weeks of electrical muscle conditioning, histological and metabolic changes take place in the transposed muscle, such as increase in the percentage of type I fatigue-resistant fibres from 46% to 64%, increased microcirculation and increased mitochondrial relative volume.[40] Electrical stimulation induces histological changes in transposed muscle and its function.[40]

Dynamic graciloplasty can be performed in two stages: stage I, graciloplasty surgery and implant of neuromuscular stimulator; stage II, conditioning of the transposed gracilis muscle. The gracilis is mobilised and the distal end is wrapped around the anal canal. It is essential that the neurovascular bundle be identified, tested and preserved for proper function of the leads and neuromuscular stimulator. The distal tendon is usually attached to the contralateral ischial tuberosity. System implantation is usually performed at the same time as the graciloplasty. Electrode placement sites are selected based on strongest muscle contraction while allowing the lowest effective stimulation settings. The stimulator is placed in a subcutaneous pocket formed in the abdomen. The muscle stimulation conditioning is usually started within 2 weeks of implantation of the system. The objective is gradually to increase stimulation time until the stimulator is programmed to continuous output after 8 weeks. After conditioning the muscle should be able to sustain prolonged contractions. The patient will be able to turn the stimulator off with an external magnet to allow defaecation.

In several studies, this new procedure has been shown to restore or improve continence in most patients. Baeten[41] performed the first successful dynamic graciloplasty procedure at the Maastricht University Hospital. In his series[42] of 52 patients, 73% were continent after a median follow-up of 2.1 years. At 52 weeks the patient's conditions had improved with respect to the median frequency of defaecation (from 5 to 2 times per 24 hours, $P<0.001$). The median time that defaecation could be postponed improved from 9 seconds to 19 minutes ($P=0.005$). Williams[43] reported 63% functioning neosphincters in 32 patients (20 incontinent patients and 12 anorectal reconstruction) treated by dynamic graciloplasty and Konsten[42] achieved 65% complete faecal continence in 26 patients who received implanted electrostimulation therapy. Seccia et al.[44] confirm that electrostimulated graciloplasty represents a reliable form of treatment for faecal incontinence and the most effective way to reconstruct the anal sphincter after surgical removal of the anorectal apparatus. In their series, 86 patients underwent a bilateral electrostimulated graciloplasty. Adopting long-term stimulation using implantable stimulators and intramuscular electrodes, continence reached 100% in patients after rectal excision and 83% in incontinent patients. Significant differences were also observed in resting and voluntary anal pressures (13.3–60.5 mmHg and 32–103 mmHg, respectively, $P<0.01$). In a recent report from the Cleveland Clinic in Florida, Wexner et al.[45] achieved an improvement in continence, social interactions and quality of life in 60% of 17 patients who underwent stimulated gracilis neosphincter operation. Manometric results showed an average basal pressure of 43 mmHg and an average maximum squeeze pressure that increased from 36 mmHg before surgery to 145 mmHg by stimulation ($P<0.01$). We have achieved an 86% success rate in treating incontinent patients. This involved revisions in three patients.

Gluteal Muscle Transfer

In patients who have lost significant muscle about the anal canal due to trauma or congenital abnormalities, an attractive alternative to the gracilis is gluteal muscle transfer. Here the gluteal muscles are used to encircle the anal canal.

Bilateral parasacral incisions are made and carried deep to the level of the gluteal muscle. The lower edge of the gluteal muscle is identified and followed outward bilaterally. Approximately 6 cm of muscle is incised from the origin of the muscle on the sacrum bilaterally, taking care not to interrupt any of the blood supply or nerve supply to the muscle during the mobilisation. It is then split in two bilaterally. There are thus four ends of muscle. These ends are then wrapped around the anus. The cranial ends of the split muscle are passed anteriorly and the more caudal ends posteriorly. This enables a scissors-like action to occur upon squeezing the gluteal muscles.

Although this is an old operation, its use has been resurrected. Pearl et al.[46] obtained good results in 4 of 7 patients and Devesa et al.[47] obtained improvement in 6 of 10 patients. Christiansen et al.[48] from University of Copenaghen treated seven patients with anal incontinence in whom previous surgery had failed by bilateral gluteus maximus transposition. All patients were incontinent to solid stool. After 1-year follow-up three patients experienced improved continence but in four incontinence was unchanged. Anorectal physiology studies showed moderately increased resting and squeeze pressures in patients who were improved by the operation. This series does not indicate that better results are obtained by gluteus transposition.

It is possible also that the results of gluteus maximus transposition could be improved by implantation of a stimulator. The chances of a successful implantation into the gluteus maximus are probably less than for the gracilis because of more variable innervation, but one successful case of stimulated gluteus maximus transposition has been reported.[48]

Role of Prostheses

Many patients with severe faecal incontinence can be successfully managed by the use of a fully implanted artificial anal sphincter. Early experience[49,50] has demonstrated that continence can be restored with acceptable morbidity. Recently we reported[51] the combined experience at the University of Minnesota and the University of Edinburgh with the use of a fully implantable artificial anal sphincter in 12 patients who failed conventional management of faecal incontinence. Careful patient follow-up was recorded during a mean 58-month follow-up. A successful outcome was achieved in nine patients (75%). Postoperative manometric studies documented establishment of an elevated high-pressure zone compared with preoperative resting pressures. Seven patients reported continence to solid stool. Two patients had some problems with control of liquid stool and three had occasional incontinence to flatus. Six of the seven patients rated their bowel control as good to excellent. Christiansen and Lorentzen[49] reported their initial experience with five patients with neurogenic incontinence. They noted that the system worked for solid or semisolid stool but less well for liquid stool. In a subsequent report on 12 patients implanted, Christiansen[50] achieved excellent results in 5, good results in 3 and acceptable results in 2. Two patients developed infection necessitating removal.

The artificial anal sphincter is a modification of the AMS 800 urinary sphincter adopted for use around the anus for faecal incontinence. It consists of three silastic parts: (1) an inflatable cuff, (2) a pressure-regulating balloon, (3) a control pump. The cuff is available in 2 to 2.5-cm widths. The pressure-regulating balloon is available in several pressure ranges varying from 60 to 90 cm of water pressure. The control pump can be activated or deactivated.

The inflatable cuff is implanted around the anus and is connected by silastic tubing to the control pump implanted in the scrotum of men and in the labia of women. The control pump is connected to the pressure-regulating balloon implanted in the space of Retzius. The system is filled with an optimum volume of fluid. In its activated state, the cuff is distended with fluid to occlude the anus and maintain continence. Cuff pressure is maintained by the pressure-regulating balloon. When the patient experiences the urge to defaecate the control pump is compressed several times, which displaces fluid out of the cuff and into the pressure-regulating balloon. This empties the cuff, thereby, decreasing anal pressure and allowing defaecation to occur. The control pump then regulates slow return of fluid from the balloon to the cuff during a 7 to 10-minute time span, thus restoring continence.

Role of Colostomy

When the surgical repairs have either failed or have no reasonable chance of succeeding, it should be remembered that a stoma will provide the patient afflicted with anal incontinence with a much better quality of life. An end-sigmoid colostomy is the preferred stoma whenever feasible. However occasionally patients will have further problems with mucus and bloody discharge due to diversion proctitis.

Summary and Conclusions

Faecal incontinence is often a multifactorial problem. All patients undergoing surgery for faecal incontinence should be fully evaluated to be sure that the degree of incontinence merits surgical intervention. The most successful of surgical treatments is sphincter reconstruction with or without levatorplasty for a disrupted anal sphincter. Post-anal repair is no longer advocated for patients with neurological damage. For severe incontinence, muscle transfers (gracilis, gluteus maximus) can achieve some success but continence is less than perfect. The development and use of an artificial anal sphincter is proceeding. For patients in whom all therapeutic options have failed, a stoma will provide a better quality of life.

References

1. Henry MM, Swash M, Phillips RKS et al. (1992) Faecal incontinence. In: Henry MM, Swash M (eds) Coloproctology and the pelvic floor, 2nd edn. Butterworth-Heinemann, Oxford, pp 257–304.
2. Farouk R, Duthie GS, MacGregor AB, Bartolo DCC (1994) Evidence of electro- mechanical dissociation of the internal anal sphincter in idiopathic fecal incontinence. Dis Colon Rectum 37:595–601.
3. Sun WM, Read NW, Miner PB, Kerrigan DD, Donelly TC (1990) The role of transient internal sphincter relaxation in faecal incontinence. Int J Colorectal Dis 5:31–36.
4. Read NW (1990) Functional assessment of the anorectum in faecal incontinence. In: Neurobiology of incontinence. Wiley, Chichester, pp 119–138 (Ciba Foundation Symposium 151).
5. Bartolo DCC, Duthie GS (1990) The physiological evaluation of operative repair for incontinence and prolapse. In: Neurobiology of incontinence. Wiley, Chichester, pp 223–245 (Ciba Foundation Symposium 151).
6. Bartolo DCC,Roe AM, Virjee J, Mortensen NJMcC (1985) Evacuation proctography in obstructed defecation and rectal intussusception. Br J Surg 72(Suppl): S111–S116.
7. Tjandra JJ,Milsom JW,Schroeder T,Fazio VW (1993) Endoluminal ultrasound is preferable to electromyography in mapping anal sphincter defects. Dis Colon Rectum 36:689–692.
8. Law PJ, Kamm MA, Bartram CI (1991) Anal endosonography in the investigation of fecal incontinence. Br J Surg 78:312–314.
9. Mann CV, Glass RE (1991) Technique of anal sphincter repair. In: Mann CV, Glass RE (eds) Surgical treatment of anal incontinence. Springer, Berlin Heidelberg New York, pp 103–106.
10. Miller NF, Brown GL (1937) The surgical treatment of complete perineal tears in the female. Am J Obstet Gynecol 34:196–209.
11. Leider S, Paskin H (1951) Post-operative traumatic anal incontinence. Ann Surg 133:240–243.
12. Blaisdell PC (1950) Plastic repair of the incontinent sphincter ani. Am J Surg 79:174–183.
13. Parks AG, McPartlin JF (1971) Late repair of injuries of the anal sphincter. Proc R Soc Med 64:1187–1189.
14. Slade MS, Goldberg SM, Schottler JL, et al. (1977) Sphincteroplasty for acquired anal inconctinence. Dis Colon Rectum 20:33–35.
15. Fang DT, Nivatvongs S, Vermeulen FD, Herman FN, Goldberg SM, Rothenberger DA (1984) Overlapping sphincteroplasty for acquired anal incontinence. Dis Colon Rectum 27:720–722.
16. Browning GGP, Motson RW (1983) Results of Parks's operation for faecal incontinence. Br Med J 286:1873–1875.
17. Keighley MRB, Fielding JWL (1983) Management of faecal incontinence and results of surgical treatment. Br J Surg 70:463–468.
18. Ctercteko GH, Fazio VW, Jagelman DG, Lavery IC, Weakley FL, Melia M (1988) Anal sphincter repair: a report of 60 cases and review of the literature. Aust NZ J Surg 58:703–710.
19. Miller R, Orrom WJ, Cornes H, Duthie GS, Bartolo DCC (1989) Anterior sphincter plication and levatorplasty in the treatment of faecal incontinence. Br J Surg 76:1058–1060.
20. Sitzler PJ, Thomson JPS (1996) Overlap repair of damaged anal sphincter: a single surgeon's series. Dis Colon Rectum 39:1356–1360.

21. Sangwan YP, Coller JA, Barrett RC et al. (1996) Unilateral pudendal neuropathy: impact on outcome of anal sphincter repair. Dis Colon Rectum 39:686–689.

22. Wexner SD, Marchetti F, Jagelman DG (1991) The role of sphincteroplasty for faecal incontinence reevaluated: a prospective physiologic and functional review. Dis Colon Rectum 34:22–30.

23. Osterberg A, Graf W, Holmberg A, Pahlman L, Ljung A, Hakelius L (1996) Long-term results of anterior levatorplasty for faecal incontinence: a retrospective study. Dis Colon Rectum 39:671–675.

24. Parks AG (1975) Anorectal incontinence. Proc R Soc Med 68:681–690.

25. Duthie GS, Bartolo DCC (1992) Faecal continence and defaecation. In: Henry MM, Swash M (eds) Coloproctology and the pelvic floor, 2nd edn. Butterworth-Heinemann, Oxford, pp 86–97.

26. Bartolo DCC, Roe AM, Locke-Edmunds JC, Virjee J, Mortensen NJMcC (1986) Flap-valve theory of anorectal incontinence. Br J Surg 73:1012–1014.

27. Miller R, Bartolo DCC, Locke-Edmunds JC, Mortensen NJMcC (1988) Prospective study of conservative and operative treatment for faecal incontinence. Br J Surg 75:101–105.

28. Orrom WJ, Miller R, Cornes H, Duthie GS, Mortensen NJMcC, Bartolo DCC (1991) Comparison of anterior sphincteroplasty and post-anal repair in the treatment of idiophatic faecal incontinence. Dis Colon Rectum 34:305–310.

29. Browning GGP, Parks AG (1983) . Post-anal repair for neuropathic faecal incontinence: correlation of clinical results and anal canal pressures. Br J Surg 70:101–104.

30. Yoshioka K, Keighley MRB (1989) Critical assessment of the quality of continence after post-anal repair for faecal incontinence. Br J Surg 76:1054–1057.

31. Womack NR, Morrison JFB, Williams NS (1988) A prospective study of the effects of post-anal repair in neurogenic faecal incontinence. Br J Surg 75:48–52.

32. Rainey JB, Donaldson DR, Thomson JPS (1990) Post-anal repair: which patients derive most benefit?. J R Coll Surg Edinb 35:101–105.

33. Yoshioka K, Hyland G, Keighley MRB (1988) Physiological changes after post-anal repair and parameters predicting outcome. Br J Surg 75:1220–1224.

34. Christiansen J, Sorensen M, Rasmussen OO (1990) Gracilis muscle transposition for faecal incontinence. Br J Surg 77:1039–1040.

35. Pickrell KL (1959) Gracilis muscle transplant for the correction of neurogenic rectal incontinence. Surg Clin North Am 39:1405.

36. Leguit P Jr, van Baal JG, Brummelkamp WH (1985) Gracilis muscle transposition in the treatment of faecal incontinence; long-term follow-up and evaluation of anal pressure recordings. Dis Colon Rectum 28:1–4.

37. Corman ML (1985) Gracilis muscle transposition for anal incontinence: late results. Br J Surg 72 (Suppl):21–22.

38. Faucheron JL, Hannoun L, Thome C, Parc R (1994) Is fecal continence improved by non-stimulated gracilis muscle transposition? Dis Colon Rectum 37:979–983.

39. Yoshioka K, Keighley MRB (1988) Clinical and manometric assessment of gracilis muscle transplant for faecal incontinence. Dis Colon Rectum 31:767–769.

40. Konsten J, Baeten CG, Havenith MG, Soeters PB (1993) Morphology of dynamic graciloplasty compared with the anal sphincter. Dis Colon Rectum 36:559–563.

41. Baeten CG, Geerdes BP, Adang EM et al.(1995) Anal dynamic graciloplasty in the treatment of intractable fecal incontinence. N Engl J Med 332:1600–1605.

42. Konsten J, Baeten CG, Spaans F, Havenith MG, Soeters PB (1993) Follow-up of anal dynamic graciloplasty for faecal incontinence. World J Surg 17:404–408.

43. Williams NS, Patel J, George BD, Hallan RI, Watkins ES (1991) Development of an electrically stimulated neoanal sphincter. Lancet 338:1166–1169.

44. Seccia M, Menconi C, Balestri R, Cavina E (1994) Study protocols and functional results in 86 electrostimulated graciloplasties. Dis Colon Rectum 37:897–904.

45. Wexner SD, Gonzalez-Padron A, Rius J, Teoh TA, Cheong DM, Nogueras JJ (1996) Stimulated gracilis neosphincter operation: initial experience, pitfalls and complications. Dis Colon Rectum 39:957–964.

46. Pearl RK, Prasad ML, Nelson RL, Orsay CP, Abcarian H (1991) Bilateral gluteus maximus transposition for anal incontinence. Dis Colon Rectum 34:478–481.

47. Devesa JM, Vicente E, Enriquez JM et al. (1992) Total fecal incontinence – a new method of gluteus maximus transposition: preliminary results and report of previous experience with similar procedures. Dis Colon Rectum 35:339–341.

48. Christiansen J, Ronholt Hansen H, Rasmussen O (1995) Bilateral gluteus maximus transposition for anal incontinence. Br J Surg 82:903–905.

49. Christiansen J, Lorentzen M (1989) Implantation of artificial sphincter for anal incontinence: report of five cases. Dis Colon Rectum 32:432–436.
50. Christiansen J, Sparso B (1992) Treatment of anal incontinence by an implantable prosthetic anal sphincter. Ann Surg 215:383–386.
51. Wong WD, Jensen LL, Bartolo DCC, Rothenberger DA (1996) Artificial anal sphincter. Dis Colon Rectum 39:1345–1351.

8 Colorectal Disease and the Law: A Surgeon's View

P.F. Schofield

Introduction

The civil justice system in the UK is in the process of change and whether the most radical elements of these changes will be modified or remain unaltered is difficult to know. In 1996 there was Lord Woolf's report on civil justice, which seeks to speed up the process of litigation and ensure that justice is widely available[1]. How these changes will impact on the colon and rectal surgeon in general and medical litigation is far from certain. Lord Woolf would like to see widening of arbitration to settle disputes with a fast track for disputes involving small potential amounts of money in damages. He has also suggested that the court should actively manage the more complex cases with a court-appointed expert. These changes have not been received with universal acclaim by the legal profession and there is justifiable doubt as to how the new system will work.

However, there is clear intention to "modernise" the civil legal system and to change the basis of legal aid, which is now effectively available to only 30% of the population. Lord Irvine, the Lord Chancellor, made his determination towards reform of legal aid clear when he said at the Solicitors' Annual Conference in October 1997:

> Civil justice is too expensive and too exclusive. The very rich and the very poor have access but middle income Britain is left in the cold and middle income Britain is the overwhelming majority of the people in this country.[2]

The Lord Chancellor asked Sir Peter Middleton to review civil justice and legal aid and he reported in September 1997.[3] It is inappropriate to go into the details of this report but it supported and enlarged on the conclusions of Lord Woolf on the reform of civil justice. The major additional proposal is in relationship to legal aid, which will not be available for cases involving damages where there is a suitable alternative form of funding. Sir Peter sees these matters being covered by conditional fees and that contingency fees should be reconsidered. The Lord Chancellor envisages that legal aid work will be restricted to providers who have a contract with the local Legal Aid Board who will administer the system as a fixed-price service.[2]

Conditional fees may be satisfactory to lawyers but they makes life uncomfortable for any expert witness in civil cases. It is important that the expert is impartial, and this appears to be the basis of Lord Woolf's court appointed expert. However, most (97%) litigation in surgical negligence cases never gets to court, and the role of the expert is to advise the solicitor and barrister on the medical aspects of the case. It is important that the expert should give a dispassionate opinion outlining both the rights and wrongs of a case. It is clear that the expert should not agree to work on a contingency basis but it is a worry that solicitors acting for the Plaintiff on a contingency basis may prefer the report which is favourable to their case even though it is biased. Are we going towards a system of "the hired gun" which some claim is prevalent in the USA?

Whilst some of the proposed changes seem alarming to doctors there are signs that many doctors would welcome Lord Woolf's emphasis on alternative dispute resolution and arbitration together with his recent statement that he sees merit in no-fault compensation.[4] Sir Peter Middleton also recommends that a further examination of the possible advantages of no-fault schemes and strict liability should be undertaken for medical negligence cases.[3]

What the future holds is difficult to predict because there are reasons to believe that litigation may become less slow and adversarial and more easily resolved by alternative dispute resolution measures or even by the introduction of no-fault compensation. However, whether litigation for medical negligence decreases or increases in the future it is important that we remain aware of the risks and try to mitigate them.

In recent years there has been an explosion in medical negligence cases in the UK and it is estimated that legally aided cases have cost the tax payer three and a half billion pounds (rising from £53 million per year to £125 million per year).[5] The medical defence societies estimate that less than one in three legally aided cases are won by the litigant.[6] However, win or lose, the defence organisations receive no costs in such cases. In turn, this means that the defence subscriptions of the doctors rise year on year. So each year the doctor may be confronted with the stress of litigation, however unjustified, as well as bearing some of the financial burden of the litigation.

In 1996 Jones[5] carried out a survey of 1559 doctors and found that a third had received a solicitor's letter and 12.7% had had proceedings issued against them. Surgeons are much more at risk than indicated by these figures. It is difficult for any surgeon to be dispassionate about any complaint alleging negligence. They feel personally involved even though in the National Health Service they do not carry financial liability since Crown Indemnity was introduced on 1 January 1990. As numbers of claims for negligence have increased in recent years, in November 1995 the National Health Service Litigation Authority (NHSLA) was started and administers the Clinical Negligence Scheme for Trusts, which acts as an insurer against claims for negligence.[4] In private practice the surgeon is at risk as the principle in any claim of negligence and has to carry increasing subscription to the defence organisation as litigation increases.

The Civil Justice System

The law recognises that it is important that matters are clearly defined. It is important that doctors understand what is required to establish proof and what is meant by legal terms in common use such as causation and quantum.

In civil cases the standard of proof required is stated as "on balance of probabilities". You will see this differs from the criminal law, which expects proof to be beyond reasonable doubt. In practice this means that in civil cases, if something is 51% probable it is accepted as fact whilst if it is 49% probable it is not accepted.

The first fundamental in medical negligence cases is to establish breach of the duty of care (liability) and this is defined by the Bolam test.[7] This arose from a judgement in 1957 in which it was stated by the judge, Mr Justice McNair:

> A medical person is not guilty of negligence if he has acted in accordance with a practice accepted as proper by a responsible body of medical men skilled in that particular art. ... Putting it the other way round, a man is not negligent if he acts in accordance with a practice, merely because there is another body of opinion who would take a contrary view.

Although the Bolam test has been challenged by some eminent legal authorities it has been little changed to this day. If a low standard of care is established, then in order to establish negligence it is necessary to show that the breach of duty of care caused harm. This is referred to as causation, that is, what is the difference between the patient's state and that which would have pertained if there had been no harm? This consideration and the prognosis is an area that has to be considered in any successful medical negligence case in order to decide on how much compensation the litigant is to receive, known as quantum.

Despite the concern about Lord Woolf's proposals the new rules for civil justice were published in January 1999 and came into effect on 26 April 1999 with the aim of speedier, more open and cheaper resolution of cases. There is an obligation on the part of the litigant (now called the Claimant) to state at the onset of the case whether the amount which is expected to be claimed for damages is more or less than £1000 which will allow allocation to the small claims court, if appropriate.

There will be two other categories, fast track for cases with damages assessed at up to £15,000 and multitrack for other cases. Most cases of personal injury other than medical negligence will fall into the fast track group and there will be an attempt to have only a single expert agreed by both Claimant and Defence. This expert will be agreed by both parties and instructed by both parties. The expert's duty will be to the Court to sort out an unbiased disinterested opinion. Either party may ask for clarification of the report by submitting questions which must be answered within 28 days. If a case goes to Court the expert will only be called to give oral evidence in exceptional cases and the Court will rely on the written medical report.

The potential medical negligence case will usually fall into the multitrack but it seems likely that the Claimant's solicitor will need medical advice before starting any action in order to assess the risks. At this time the situation is less clear because although the rules for experts have been set out, the protocol for experts is not completed. There seems little doubt that in these complex cases more than one expert will be required but that the information in the reports will be disclosed much earlier than has been the case in the past. As part of this openness, meetings of experts will be encouraged in order to inform the Court where there is agreement and disagreement and why there is disagreement.

Finally it is emphasized in Rule 35 that the expert's duty is to the Court, not to the person who has instructed or paid the expert.

The Medical Expert

Anyone agreeing to be a medical expert should accept that this may be time-consuming and may interfere with clinical practice. In addition to the report writing you may have to attend case conferences and appear in court. The latter is not likely as 97% of cases are settled out of court but it can be disruptive if it is necessary to spend several days in court or even more likely to be booked for court and be told at a few days notice that the case is settled. One of Lord Woolf's recommendations is to minimise the time spent in court by the doctor.

If you are willing to act it is important that you only agree to be an expert in areas in which you are completely at home. It is equally important that you can express your expertise in a fashion which will be understood by an "intelligent layman", in particular by a judge. To do this requires experience but most importantly it requires training. Not only should the medical expert be expert in the field but he must be able to communicate that expertise in a readily accessible form in a written report and be prepared to defend his opinion in a court of law.

The expert witness has been long accepted in legal matters. The modern role was defined more than two centuries ago when it was agreed that an accepted expert could give an opinion based on the facts.[9] In that case the expert was a Mr Smeaton, a eminent engineer, who was called by the defendants in an action which involved the effects of the demolition of a sea bank on a harbour. There was dispute as to whether his evidence was admissible as it was based on opinion. The learned judge, Lord Mansfield, said.

> It is objected, that Mr Smeaton is going to speak, not to the facts, but as to opinion. That opinion, however, is deduced from the facts which, are not disputed. ... The cause of the decay of the harbour is also a matter of science, and still more so, whether the removal of the bank can be judged beneficial. Of this, such men as Mr Smeaton alone can judge. Therefore, we are of the opinion that his judgement, formed on the facts, was proper evidence".

Thus the first expert was allowed to speak and give opinion to the court. This placed the expert in a unique position because the expert alone was permitted to give opinion but this opinion does not need to be accepted by the court.

The areas in which a colorectal surgeon may be expected to act as an expert would usually involve civil cases principally and rarely involve criminal cases. The civil cases may arise from an accidental injury or an injury from alleged medical negligence.

Accidental Injury

The coloproctologist is rarely asked for an opinion regarding accidents because most of the work falls into the province of the orthopaedic surgeon. However, there are a few issues where an opinion may be requested because for most surgeons engaged in coloproctology their area of expertise would cover abdominal injuries and hernias as well bowel disease.

Hernia

The reason surgeons are asked about hernia is in relationship to injury at work because it is recognised that hernia may be traumatic. What is less well recognised is that most hernias cannot be attributed to a strain.[10] Most courts will accept that a hernia is due to trauma if:

(a) There is a history of a sudden strain
(b) There is groin pain at the time
(c) The incident is reported at work
(d) The diagnosis of hernia is made shortly after the incident.[11]

In terms of disability after hernia repair it is still poorly recognised that recurrence of the hernia is no more likely on returning to heavy manual work than returning to a sedentary occupation[12] and a satisfactorily repaired hernia is not a disadvantage in the job market.[13]

Complications of Hernia Repair

These may lead to a medical negligence claim. The principal problems are persisting pain and testicular atrophy. Some discomfort in the groin lasting for weeks is not uncommon after hernia repair but it usually settles spontaneously provided there is no recurrence of the hernia. Persisting pain not due to recurrence can be a considerable problem after hernia repair, not least because it is recognised that pain may be due to ilioinguinal or genitofemoral nerve entrapment[14] and in laparoscopic hernia repair entrapment of the lateral cutaneous nerve of thigh.[15]

In my experience, many cases are given the label nerve entrapment when this is not the cause of the pain. The term nerve entrapment is unfortunate because it can be perceived by lawyers to mean that the nerve has become entrapped due to a negligent act. Further problems may arise when the diagnosis of nerve pain is illogically maintained despite the fact that appropriate nerve blocks have had no effect on the pain. Most patients with pain after a hernia repair do not have nerve entrapment but the exact cause of the persisting pain in this group of patients is difficult to establish.[16] It may be due to muscle strain, to deafferentation, which can affect any wound, or it may be psychological or it may be malingering. Complaint of wound pain, whatever the cause, is rarely judged to be due to negligence.

Testicular atrophy is a rare but recognised complication of hernia repair which is not necessarily due to negligence. It has an incidence which lies between 0.03% and 0.5% after a primary inguinal hernia repair and this hazard is not usually discussed with the patient.[17] The incidence is significantly higher in recurrent hernia and it is recommended in the Royal College of Surgeons of England guidelines that warnings of the risk of testicular atrophy should be given for operation for repair of recurrent hernia or scrotal hernia or after previous vasectomy.[18] The testicular problem probably arises from venous thrombosis in the pampiniform plexus which causes testicular venous congestion with swelling rather than arterial thrombosis.[19] The swelling frequently settles without long-term damage but may lead to venous necrosis of the testis with subsequent testicular atrophy. It should be possible to mount a successful defence against an action brought for negligence regarding testicular atrophy after a primary hernia repair.

Abdominal Injury

The aspect of general injury work that the coloproctologist is most asked about concerns abdominal injuries. Often these are part of multiple injuries so that an orthopaedic surgeon or a neurosurgeon may also be producing reports. In these cases, it is important to indicate in your report that you will deal with the abdominal injury alone and that others will deal with the other injuries.

As far as the immediate impact of the injuries is concerned, this is important because of the effect on pain and suffering but in general the more important elements of an abdominal injury are the medium- and long-term consequences of the injury. Resection of bowel is rarely so great as to produce persistent diarrhoea or potential metabolic problems but the possibility should be kept in mind when assessing the operation note and when assessing the patient. The creation of a colostomy is seen as a significant disability and its effects need to be spelt out.

Splenectomy does carry significant risks of overwhelming infection in children and in adults with haematological disease but the risks are small in fit adults.[20] The infections are most commonly due to *Streptococcus pneumoniae*. The other two principal causative organisms are *Haemophilus influenzae* and *Neisseria meningitidis*. The infection rate is at the greatest in infants where it is recorded as occurring in 15.7% of cases. The frequency of infection in children under 16 years is 4.4% with a mortality of 2.2%. By contrast, adults who are otherwise normal do not appear to have an increased frequency of infection. The pattern of infection differs between children and adults. In young children it is more likely to be a meningitis whilst in adults it is usually an overwhelming septicaemia.[20] It is recommended that all asplenic patients should have vaccination against *S. pneumoniae* by Pneumovax II and that vaccination against *H. influenzae* type b (Hib) and *N. meningitidis* types A and C should be performed. The Chief Medical Officer recommends that for children under 16 years of age a regular prophylactic antibiotic should also be given (penicillin V twice daily has been suggested).[21]

Disruption of work and social activity caused by the injury are to be considered as well as persisting symptoms and future risks. The abdominal scar, although sound, may be considered a disfigurement, especially in a female. A weakness of a vertical scar may be present or may develop in the future. Less than half of the incisional hernias that develop are apparent 1 year after operation.[22] An instance of 4% at 2 years after operation has been quoted by Condon[23] and the Oxford textbook of surgery suggests that the rate of herniation may increase to 10% with long-term follow up.[24]

The most important long-term risk is that of small bowel obstruction due to adhesions. Although this risk is not great it should be documented after any abdominal operation. It has been suggested that the risk is about 3–4% after any laparotomy of which a third occur in the first year after operation, a little less than a third at 1–5 years and a little more than a third after 5 years.[25] It is recognised that the risk of adhesion obstruction is greater after pelvic or colonic surgery.[26]

Stress and Infection and Inflammatory Bowel Disease

The possibility that an injury or an infection may produce or worsen inflammatory bowel disease (IBD) is an issue which may require an opinion from a colorectal expert in cases involving an accident. A small proportion of previously healthy patients develop an infective colitis that does not resolve and the clinical picture changes to typical ulcerative colitis. In those cases it seems that the infection unmasks or causes the ulcerative colitis.[27] Similar progression from infective colitis to Crohn's disease has been reported. These issues become of legal importance when the initial bowel infection is due to the possible negligence of an hotel or caterer. McKendrick and Read[28] studied 38 patients after an outbreak of food poisoning due to *Salmonella enteritidis.* Twelve of these patients continued to have symptoms of bowel irritation for 12 months after the infection had settled. They felt these patients had irritable bowel syndrome but none developed IBD. A subsequent study with 540 patients indicated that a quarter of them had persistence of altered bowel habit 6 months after the resolution of an episode of gastroenteritis.[29] None of these patients developed IBD but, whilst some had preexisting bowel symptoms, about 7% met the criteria for new irritable bowel syndrome.

There is little or no evidence that injury or stress causes inflammatory bowel disease although it may worsen the symptoms temporarily.[30] The course and prognosis of inflammatory bowel disease is rarely relevant in the medicolegal area but it can cause problems for the sufferer to get life insurance. In the UK about 70% of insurance companies either refuse to give patients cover or offer policies with very heavy weighting.[31] When it is known that at any time about 90% of patients with ulcerative colitis will be working and 90% will still be working in 10 years time it seems harsh to refuse insurance cover. The position is only a little less optimistic for patients with Crohn's disease but recent studies show that the majority of patients are able to work full time.[32] In particular, not only the working capacity but also the life expectancy of patients with IBD is much better than has been generally accepted.

Medical Negligence

Medical negligence costs began to rise rapidly in the USA from the late 1960s and continue to rise progressively.[33] In the UK we were fortunate that good doctor–patient relationships prevented this early explosion of litigation but times have changed and medical negligence costs are rising rapidly. In 1992–1993, the cost of claims was £80 million but in 1994–1995 it was £125 million.[34]

In the USA general surgery ranks second in the list of both claims and costs only after obstetrics and gynaecology.[35] Colorectal disease was moderately high amongst the causes of litigation but most of the cases were against internists or general surgeons; specialist colorectal surgeons were amongst the least involved in litigation, indeed they were involved in only 3% of cases of negligence involving colon and rectal disease. It is interesting to see that female breast disease was the most common cause of litigation; hernia repair, appendicitis and biliary surgery were almost as common but colon and rectal disease is less likely to be the cause of litigation.

However, little was known about the causes of litigation involving colon and rectal disease until the past few years. The data largely comes from the USA but seems to be in agreement with cases which have presented to me. Kern[33] indicates that there are five main categories into which allegations fall. In order of frequency they are:

- Diagnostic delay, usually of cancer
- Colon injury
- Complications of treatment or investigation
- Anal injury leading to incontinence
- Lack of informed consent.

Coloproctologists may be involved in the management of two types of case that can lead to action for negligence:

- Injuries to the bowel or anus caused by other doctors
- Inadequate management by the coloproctologist.

Faecal Incontinence

The commonest cause of faecal incontinence is childbirth injury. The other important cause of incontinence is anal surgery.

Childbirth Injury

The work of Sultan and colleagues[36,37] has exposed how frequently anal sphincter injury occurs during childbirth and how ignorant the average midwife and the average senior house officer is of perineal anatomy. The situation becomes critical with tears in childbirth that involve the anal canal (It is best to avoid the term third-degree tear because there is no agreement about the definition.) Full documentation of the findings and the technique of repair are essential. If an anal involvement is not recognised or the repair is not well documented it is difficult to defend an allegation of negligence when faecal incontinence develops subsequently.

A further study by Sultan et al.[38] investigated the results of primary repairs of childbirth injuries involving the anal sphincter. This study indicated that the results of primary repair were not as good as previously thought. However, the assessments were made only 6 weeks after delivery in only 34 women, which is too small a group to draw wide-ranging conclusions. In my view, a more sound recent paper on primary repair came from Colchester where 81 patients were assessed 3 months after childbirth complicated by the repair of a "third-degree" tear.[39] In this study 80% of patients had complete continence, 12% had defective control of flatus and 7% had faecal incontinence. These results contrast sharply with the figures quoted by Sultan et al.[38]

Delayed repair for incontinence several months after anal sphincter injury does not appear to give as satisfactory results as primary repair. A recent study of delayed repair indicated that 45% achieved complete continence, 31% still had defective control of flatus and 20% remained faecally incontinent after repair.[40]

Anal Surgery

The other major cause of faecal incontinence is anal incontinence is anal surgery and this can occur after any type of anal procedure. It is particularly true of operations to eliminate a fistula-in-ano, even a low fistula-in-ano. The degree of altered continence may be occasional soiling, incontinence of flatus or true faecal incontinence. The risk is higher in an anterior fistula in females or when the fistula has a high extension or is trans-sphincteric. Even after operation for a low fistula there may be some degree of impaired continence. One study indicated that minor incontinence occurred in about a quarter of the patients and significant faecal incontinence in 7% of patients.[41]

After anal dilatation, whether for fissure or for another indication, there is an incidence of incontinence. Forcible anal dilatation may produce serious internal anal sphincter disruption leading to persistent faecal seepage.[42] For this reason lateral anal internal sphincterotomy was the treatment of choice for chronic anal fissure until recently, yet even after this procedure there was evidence of faecal seepage in about 6% of patients, which persisted for more than 6 weeks[43]

Haemorrhoidectomy is not immune from the complication of incontinence because there are examples of internal anal sphincter damage associated with this operation leading to incontinent seepage of faecal material. Finally, even minor procedures for haemorrhoids can produce complications. Elastic band ligation (EBL) may produce severe but transitory pain but on very rare occasions it has been complicated by gross sepsis that has even been fatal.[44] Injection of piles with phenol in almond oil has been used for many years but misplaced injections can cause significant problems.[45] Usually a misplaced injection is made into the prostate gland leading to haematuria and dysuria. This commonly settles without long-term sequelae but it may go on to produce urethral stricture.

Colonoscopic Injury

Injury to the colon during colonoscopy may be caused by coloproctologists but many cases occur in the hands of inexperienced trainees or general physicians. The American Society of Gastrointestinal Endoscopy recognises that at least 100 procedures should be undertaken under supervision in training before independent practice can be authorised.[46]

The major risks of colonoscopy are perforation or bleeding. Perforation is more likely if a polyp has been removed. Since perforation and bleeding are rare but recognised risks of the procedure it is best to ensure that warnings are given of these risks when consent is given by the patient.

The incidence of perforation during diagnostic colonoscopy has been reported in the range of 0.03–0.67% and during therapeutic colonoscopy 0.073–2.14%.[47] There is some evidence that the frequency of this complication declines with experience.[48] It is important to recognise the possibility of free perforation quickly. However, the signs and symptoms are very variable depending on the size and site of the perforation. The symptoms may be immediate but may be delayed for many hours or days. The usual symptom is the onset of persisting abdominal pain with signs of peritoneal irritation on examination. Abdominal and chest radiography may show free intraperitoneal gas.

The management of colonoscopic perforations is not clear-cut because it has been shown that some patients will settle on non-operative management with bowel rest and antibiotics. Christie and Marrazzo[49] conclude that non-operative management was indicated if the patient's general condition remained stable without signs of spreading peritonitis even though there was free gas on X-ray. Occasionally patients develop the so-called post-polypectomy coagulation syndrome with abdominal pain and a low-grade fever developing a few hours after a polypectomy.[50] This is due to a thermal injury to the colonic wall. These patients usually recover within a few days with conservative measures. There is no doubt that operation without delay is indicated if there are general or increasing abdominal signs or adverse changes in the patient's general condition.[47] There are still some reports of rectosigmoid perforations caused by rigid sigmoidoscopy but these are considerably rarer than those with colonoscopy.[51]

Colonic haemorrhage is a very rare complication of diagnostic colonoscopy but is more likely in association with polypectomy.[48,52] It can occur either during the procedure or within days of the polypectomy. Immediate bleeding occurs because there has been inadequate coagulation of the blood vessels at the neck of the polyp whereas delayed bleeding is a secondary haemorrhage due to slough separating at the coagulation site. If immediate bleeding cannot be controlled endoscopically laparotomy is indicated to control the bleeding. Delayed bleeding rarely requires operation.

Other complications of colonoscopy are all rare, although intracolonic gas explosion has been reported but can be prevented by carbon dioxide insufflation. Cardiac irregularities have been described so monitoring is desirable. There are examples of bacteraemia and rarely septicaemia induced by colonoscopy. Because of the possibility of bacteraemia it is important that prophylactic antibiotics are given if the patient has any foreign prostatic material or heart disease.[48]

Barium Enema Perforation

Although less well documented than endoscopic perforation, barium enema has been recorded as producing both colon and rectal injury. The incidence is low but is quoted as 0.2–0.4%.[53] The condition is painful and requires urgent operation unless the perforation is extraperitoneal and small. It has been suggested that previous biopsy may predispose to perforation. Recent work suggests there is no increased risk after colonoscopic biopsies as they are superficial but there should be a few days delay after biopsy through a rigid sigmoidoscopy because such biopsies are deeper.[54]

Injuries at Open Surgery

Another potential cause of litigation is when the rectum or other area of bowel is injured by a surgeon operating in the pelvis. This is not always noticed so that peritonitis or faecal fistula may develop. Such cases are difficult to defend.

Significant colonic injury may occur in difficult dissection near the colon or rectum so that both gynaecological operations and urological operations carry the risks of large bowel damage leading to peritonitis or faecal fistula. Morse et al.[55] reported on a variety of colonic injuries associated with urological surgery. Not only did the injuries occur from pelvic surgery but they also mention two cases with colonic injury after nephrectomy.

Perineal operations may be a source of bowel damage. Small bowel or colon may be injured after uterine curettage especially in the pregnant uterus because the uterine wall is easily perforated at this time.[56] Urologists who practice radical prostatectomy indicate that there is a significant risk of bowel injury with an incidence of 0.5–3%.[57]

Minimal Invasive Procedures

Laparoscopy is a well recognised cause of bowel injury. Fortunately this complication is rare being variously quoted as 0.06–0.3% of cases.[58] These rates come from laparoscopy for gynaecological indications rather than from laparoscopy for cholecystectomy but bowel injury is recorded after laparoscopic cholecystectomy with an incidence of 0.14%.[59] The injury is usually caused by the Veress needle and is self-sealing but may be caused by a trochar when the defect needs to be repaired. Of more worrying significance is the bowel injury which is not recognised and presents after hours or days with peritonitis. This may be due to diathermy injury to the bowel rather than a missed trochar injury.[59]

Colonic injuries have been reported in percutaneous nephrolithotomy in between 0.2 and 0.5% of cases.[60] The injuries can usually be managed conservatively. Transurethral prostatectomy is a rare cause of fistula to the rectum due to injury.[55]

Radiotherapy

Radiotherapy for treatment of carcinoma cervix in particular and to a lesser extent carcinoma of the bladder, prostate and rectum may produce significant injury to the bowel, in particular the rectum, sigmoid colon and terminal ileum. The symptoms do not appear for months but may cause intestinal obstruction, rectovaginal fistula or rectal bleeding.[61] It has been realised that the hazard of delayed bowel injury is relatively high developing in 1–20% of cases after radiotherapy for carcinoma of the cervix.[62] In most centres the complication is at the lower end of this range but warnings of the risk must be given. It seems probable that there are a significant number of patients in the UK with radiation injury several of whom are seeking to take action against health authorities for damages.

Informed Consent

In coloproctology it is important to recognise the importance of informed consent and to warn of any likely complication. Many surgeons have reasoned that it is unnecessary or even unwise to warn about rare complications and as a rule of thumb it was considered that if a complication occurred less than one per

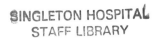

cent of the time then warnings were not required. This was overturned in the case of Smith versus Tunbridge Wells Health Authority.[63]

The case involved a young man who had an operation for rectal prolapse and subsequently developed both bladder dysfunction and impotence. Expert evidence was given that these complications were so rare that it was not necessary to give warnings about them even though they were recognised complications of the operation. Mr Justice Morehead found that although the complications were rare the litigant should have been warned because the effects were so devastating to a young man. For this reason the judgement was given in favour of the litigant. Subsequent to this judgement it has become imperative to warn all men of the risk of bladder and sexual problems in surgery requiring dissection in the pelvis.

This case will have delighted some academic lawyers who believe that the Bolam test is unreasonable because it gives too much weight to the opinion of doctors, in effect allowing the defendant's professional colleagues to usurp the function of the court in determining what is negligence.[8] Fortunately the general principle of the Bolam test, if a little modified, is still taken as the yardstick of reasonable professional behaviour.

It is of interest that fewer cases are brought in the UK because of lack of informed consent than in the USA.[33] In the UK it is acknowledged at the moment that warning of risk has to be a balance between what a reasonable patient may want to know and the raising of unreasonable fears.[64]

Pelvic Nerve Injury

The fact that impairment of sexual function including impotence and retrograde ejaculation may occur in men after pelvic surgery has been discussed above.[65]

Diagnostic Delay

When a diagnosis is delayed due to failure to take steps in the investigation of a patient there are a number of issues raised:

- Was there indication to take further steps?
- Did the delay cause harm?

The first issue is usually apparent but the issue of whether harm was caused is much more difficult to assess and may raise questions that are impossible to answer, especially in tumour cases, for example:

- How long have liver secondaries been present before they grow to diagnosable size?
- How long is an adenoma present before it changes to a carcinoma of the colon?

While there is some evidence to answer these questions it is impossible to translate the general to the specific case because all biological properties vary; the law and courts are reluctant to understand this problem, however. The result in my experience is that too great a weight is given to delay in worsening the prognosis of a tumour with serious consequences for the defendant.

The other condition which is associated with allegation of negligent delay is appendicitis. This is of particular concern in young girls and women because it may be coupled with the allegation that the delay in diagnosis has led to tubal blockage.[66] It is particularly relevant that these cases may be commenced many years after the illness because they do not fall out of time because the normal 3 year barrier does not apply to children and may not apply in young women who only become aware of their infertility at a later stage.

Ureteric Injury

Injuries to the ureter may occur in pelvic surgery. Although gynaecologists have long had worries about this type of injury associated with hysterectomy, colorectal surgeons undertaking major surgery have to be aware of the risk of ureteric damage.[67] If the injury is recognised and corrected then litigation is less likely to be successful, especially if the pelvic operation has been difficult. The literature suggests that ureteric injury occurs in between 1 in 300–400 hysterectomies.[68] The situation when the ureteric injury is not noted at operation but comes to light in the postoperative period due to urine leakage or ureteric obstruction with pain is more difficult to defend. A recent case of ureteric obstruction which was found to be due to negligence has had the judgement overturned on appeal because it was agreed that the ureteric obstruction was not necessarily due to defective technique.[68] The cases when delayed leakage has occurred are even less certain to be accepted as non-negligent. Recent cases indicate that the probable outcome in such cases is that the litigant will succeed.[68] Whilst in straightforward cases this presumption of negligence is not unreasonable, I question the validity in cases where the leakage is delayed. There is no doubt that in difficult cases, when extensive dissection is required to safeguard the ureter, its blood supply may be imperilled leading to late sloughing in some cases in which no negligence is present. There is a danger of the courts applying the doctrine of res ipsa loquitur (it speaks for itself) to all cases of ureteric injury not recognised at surgery.[69]

The Compartment Syndrome

Colorectal surgeons share with urologists and gynaecologists the requirement for operating in the pelvis. Some of these operations are very long and take place with the patient's legs raised in Lloyd-Davies supports or similar appliances. In urological and gynaecological literature, the possibility of problems with the legs occurring after a period of protracted elevation has been recognised for some years.[70] However, it has only been in recent times, especially with the introduction of ileoanal pouch surgery, that colorectal surgeons have carried out lengthy operations with the patient's legs elevated.

Compartment syndrome is a condition in which swelling occurs in an inexpansile fibro-osseous space with increasing pressure in that space which causes a reduction in perfusion pressure in the compartment. This leads to tissue necrosis, further swelling and reperfusion injury. This causes permanent loss of neuromuscular tissue unless the condition is corrected by urgent fasciotomy.

The first case of this complication after surgery for an ileoanal pouch was described in 1989.[71] The following year a report of 11 patients who underwent prolonged leg elevation during ileoanal pouch construction indicated that there was pain and swelling in the legs in four patients but they recovered without neuromuscular impairment.[72] Pressures were measured and shown to be increased in two patients but the pressure did not reach critical levels. The risks of leg elevation were brought to general attention by an article by Peters et al.[73] in 1994 when the literature was reviewed and two cases of compartment syndrome after colonic surgery were reported. In addition they studied compartment pressures in 10 volunteers. They concluded that all cases with leg elevation for more than 5 hours were at risk, and that perfusion in the compartments could be improved by reversing the head-down tilt of the operating table. It is desirable in all protracted pelvic operations to do this and if possible take the legs down in order to allow recovery after 3–4 hours of operating.

It seems possible to defend cases that occurred before 1994 because the complication was not common knowledge at that time but occurrence of this problem now would be considered negligent.

Postoperative Complications

Problems due to bleeding, anastomotic dehiscence and peritonitis may occur after a correctly performed operation. In my experience, these complications become difficult to defend if the clinical notes and the documentation of the patient monitoring is poor. The problem in these cases is that appropriate steps are not taken promptly in order to deal with the complication. The allegation of unreasonable delay cannot be countered unless there are excellent notes to support the management policy used in the individual case.

The problem is complicated by the fact that it frequently occurs "out of hours" when management may be in the hands of a relatively inexperienced surgeon who misassesses the situation, reacts inappropriately and doesn't call for experienced assistance. The inexperience of the doctor will not be accepted as a defence because a court would hold that it is the responsibility of the employing authority to ensure that there is an adequate level of expertise at all times.[74]

The development of postoperative peritonitis is a particularly difficult diagnostic problem because these patients do not have the typical features of peritonitis. The usual presentation is with obvious shortness of breath and a rapid respiratory rate with little emphasis on abdominal pain. There will be a rapid pulse and a falling blood pressure. The surgical tyro inevitably misdiagnoses the condition as being due to a pulmonary or cardiac cause. The diagnosis can be made when there is an awareness that this type of problem occurring suddenly 4–7 days after a colonic anastomosis is almost certainly due to anastomotic dehiscence. If re-operation is delayed then the mortality risk increases by the hour and such delays in re-operating have led to successful litigation claims.

Errors due to delay in the treatment of postoperative bleeding may occur but are less common. The development of tachycardia with a falling blood pressure soon after an operation is usually recognised as being due to bleeding. The patient is resuscitated by appropriate transfusion and should go on to reoperation. Occasionally after resuscitation there is a reluctance to reoperate, which can lead to either death or a protracted and difficult illness.

Wound Healing

Wound infection and wound sinuses may occur after any abdominal operation and can usually be defended against charges of negligence provided a reasonable prophylactic antibiotic regime was used at the time of operation.[75] Wound dehiscence or disruption is rare at a little under 1% and cannot be shown to be due to negligence provided an acceptable technique was used and documented.[76] The question of the wound scar, wound hernia and peritoneal adhesions have been discussed elsewhere.

Deep Vein Thrombosis and Pulmonary Embolus

An important risk after operation is the development of venous thrombosis in the legs and possible pulmonary embolism. In general the patients may be placed into three risk groups, low risk, moderate risk and high risk.[77] Low risk is minor surgery taking less than 30 minutes or major surgery in otherwise fit individuals who are less than 40 years of age. The risk of symptomatic venous thrombosis and pulmonary embolism is very low and no preventive treatment other than leg supports and early mobilisatison is required. The moderate-risk group has a more clearly defined risk of symptomatic leg vein thrombosis but a low pulmonary embolus rate. These are patients undergoing major surgery who are more than 40 years of age or who have coincidental major medical illness. It is argued that this group should have low dose heparin as a prophylaxis but there is a minority body of opinion who would rely on either compression stockings or intermittent calf compression during and after the operation. The high-risk group is those patients who require major pelvic surgery for malignancy. These patients have a high incidence of symptomatic leg vein thrombosis and pulmonary embolus, which is said to be fatal in approximately 1% of cases. Although heparin will not eliminate pulmonary embolus in this group it will reduce it, so low-dose heparin is justified.[77,78] It is important to realise that whilst there may be a reduction in deep vein thrombosis in cases given heparin, no method completely removes this risk. The dose of heparin has to be carefully controlled because doses in excess of 5000 units have a significant risk of increasing operative and postoperative haemorrhage. Recently there has been a suggestion that low molecular weight heparin carries less risk of bleeding and gives better control.[79]

Indefensible Errors

It is clear that there are some errors which are indefensible. These include operating on the wrong side, causing burns after igniting spirit preparation to the perineum and inadvertently leaving swabs or instruments inside a patient at laparotomy.[80]

Conclusion

How has the response to the increase in litigation affected the care of patients? One can observe changes which have occurred in the USA, some of which are good but some are undoubtedly bad.[81] The good effects have been to persuade physicians to keep more detailed records, to give more information to the patient and to develop written information leaflets. However, there have been bad effects producing defensive medicine defined by McQuade[82] as: "ordering of treatment, tests and procedures for the purpose of protecting the doctor from criticism rather than diagnosing or treating the patient". Further problems recorded in the USA were that physicians and surgeons refused to take high-risk cases. Finally, the cost of litigation deflects money away from patient care within the NHS. Whether Lord Woolf's hope of more arbitration and less confrontation becomes a reality is conjectural. It is encouraging that the Middleton Report[3] supports Lord Woolf's recent suggestion of further examination of no-fault compensation for injury including injury due to medical negligence.[4] I am not optimistic of such a radical change in the near future.

Clearly surgeons must accept they work in a world where confrontation is common and respect becoming rarer. The best protection against litigation comes from spending time in good patient contact, giving adequate information and writing detailed notes about the patient's treatment and progress. It cannot be stressed too highly that the surgeon must take time and trouble to communicate without using jargon and if some complication occurs explain it in simple language. I have deliberately not mentioned a high standard of medicine. We should all strive for this but without patient understanding the highest quality of medical care may be criticised. Even though such cases will ultimately fail to demonstrate negligence they cause stress for both patient and surgeon. In addition they may cause a significant financial cost before the case is settled.

Finally we must recognise that with restricted duty hours for junior staff much of the continuity of care falls on the consultant. If consultants are away for a day or the weekend, they must let the duty surgical team know about ongoing or unresolved problems. Management errors do occur because of inadequate communication between colleagues. Much of the skill in risk limitation is to be a good communicator, not only to your patient but to their relatives and your colleagues.

References

1. Lord Woolf (1996) Access to justice: final report by the Right Honourable the Lord Woolf, Master of the Rolls. HMSO, London.
2. Lord Irvine of Lairg (1997) Civil justice and legal aid reforms. Keynote address by the Lord Chancellor to the Solicitors' Annual Conference, 18 October 1997.
3. Middleton P (1997) Review of civil justice and legal aid – report to the Lord Chancellor. Lord Chancellor's Department, London.
4. Lord Woolf (1997) The medical profession and justice. J R Soc Med 90:364–367.
5. Jones MA (1996) Medical negligence, 2nd edn. Sweet and Maxwell, London.
6. Holland M (1997) Lawyers target GP errors. Medical Monitor (May):8–11.
7. Bolam v. Friern Hospital Management Committee (1957) 2 All ER 118; 1 WLR 582.
8. Harpwood V (1994) NHS reform, audit protocols and standard of care. Med Law Int 1:241–259.
9. Folkes v. Chard (1782) 3 Doug. KB 157.

10. Smith GD, Lewis PA, Crosby DL (1996) Inguinal hernia and a single strenuous event. Ann R Coll Surg Engl 78:367–368.
11. Ehrhardt ME, Fish R (1995) Medicolegal aspects of hernia. In: Nyhus LM; Condon RE (eds) Hernia, 4th edn. Lippincott, Philadelphia, pp 577–590.
12. Ross APJ (1975) Incidence of inguinal hernia recurrence. Ann R Coll Surg Engl 57:326–328.
13. Rider MA, Baker DM, Locker A, Fawcett AN (1993) Return to work after inguinal hernia repair. Br J Surg 80:745–746.
14. Starling JR, Harms BA (1989) Diagnosis and treatment of genitofemoral and ilioinguinal neuralgia. World J Surg 13:586–591.
15. Phillips EH, Arregui M, Carroll BJ et al. (1995) Incidence of complications following laparoscopic hernioplasty. Surg Endosc 9:16–21.
16. Wantz GE (1984) Complications of inguinal hernia repair. Surg Clin North Am 64:287–298.
17. Reid I, Devlin HB (1994) Testicular atrophy as a consequence of inguinal hernia repair. Br J Surg 81:91–93.
18. Report of Working Party convened by the Royal College of Surgeons of England (1993) Clinical guidelines on the management of groin hernia in adults. Royal College of Surgeons of England, London.
19. Wantz GE (1993) Testicular atrophy and chronic residual neuralgia as risks of inguinal hernioplasty. Surg Clin North Am 73:571–581.
20. Holdsworth RJ, Irving AD, Cuschieri A (1991) Postsplenectomy sepsis and its mortality rate: actual versus perceived risks. Br J Surg 78:1031–1038.
21. Department of Health (1994) Asplenic patients and immunisation. CMO's Update 1:3.
22. Ellis H, Gajraj H, George CD (1983) Incisional hernias: when do they occur? Br J Surg 70:290–291.
23. Condon RE (1995) Incisional hernia. In: Nyhus LM, Condon RE (eds) Hernia, 4th edn. Lippincott, Philadelphia pp 319–336.
24. Savage A, Lamont PM (1994) Incisional hernia including parastomal hernia. In: Morris PJ, Malt RA (eds) Oxford textbook of surgery. Oxford University Press, New York, pp 1412–1417.
25. Menzies D (1993) Postoperative adhesions: their treatment and relevance in clinical practice. Ann R Coll Surg Engl 75:147–153.
26. Menzies D, Ellis H (1990) Intestinal obstruction from adhesions – how big is the problem? Ann R Coll Surg Engl 72:60–63.
27. Wright CL, Riddell RH (1997) Acute infectious colitis – diagnostic dilemma. In: Allan AN et al. (eds) Inflammatory bowel diseases, 3rd edn. Churchill Livingstone, Edinburgh, pp. 359–368.
28. McKendrick MW, Read NW (1994) Irritable bowel syndrome – post-salmonella infection. J Infect 29:1–3.
29. Neal KR, Hebden J, Spiller R (1997) Prevalence of gastrointestinal symptoms six months after bacterial gastroenteritis and risk factors for devlopment of irritable bowel syndrome: postal survey of patients. Br Med J 314:779–782.
30. North CS, Clouse RE, Spitznagel EL, Alpers DH (1990) The relation of ulcerative colitis to psychiatric factors: a review of findings and methods. Am J Psychiatr 147:974–981.
31. Moody G, Mayberry JF (1997) Social consequences of inflammatory bowel disease. In: Allan RN et al. (eds) Inflammatory bowel diseases, 3rd edn. Churchill Livingstone, Edinburgh, pp 947–949.
32. Travis SPL (1997) Insurance risks for patients with ulcerative colitis or Crohn's disease. Aliment Pharmacol Ther 11:51–59.
33. Kern KA (1993) Medical malpractice involving colon and rectal disease: a 20-year review of United States civil court litigation. Dis Colon Rectum 36:531–539.
34. Dyer C (1996) Medical litigation faces British revolution. Br Med J 312:330.
35. Kern KA (1995) The anatomy of surgical malpractice claims. Bull Am Coll Surg 80:35–49.
36. Sultan AH, Kamm MA, Hudson CN, Thomas JM, Bartram CI (1993) Anal-sphincter disruption during vaginal delivery. N Engl J Med 329:1905–1911.
37. Sultan AH, Kamm MA, Hudson CN (1995) Obstetric perineal trauma: an audit of training. J Obstet Gynecol 15:19–23.
38. Sultan AH, Kamm MA, Hudson CN, Bartram CI (1994) Third degree obstetric anal sphincter tears: risk factors and outcome of primary repair. Br Med J 308:887–891.
39. Walsh CJ, Mooney EF, Upton GJ, Motson RW (1996) Incidence of third-degree perineal tears in labour and outcome after primary repair. Br J Surg 83:218–221.
40. Engel AF, Kamm MA, Sultan AH, Bartram CI, Nicholls RJ (1994) Anterior anal sphincter repair in patients with obstetric trauma. Br J Surg. 81:1331–334.
41. Marks CG, Ritchie JK (1977) Anal fistula at St Mark's Hospital. Br J Surg 64:84–91.
42. Speakman CTM, Burnett STD, Kamm MA, Bartram CI (1991) Sphincter injury after anal dilatation demonstrated by anal endosonography. Br J Surg 78:1429–1430.

43. Lewis TH, Corman ML, Prager ED, Robertson WG (1988) Long-term results of open and closed sphincterotomy for anal fissure. Dis Colon Rectum 31:368–371.
44. Russel TR, Donohue JH (1985) Hemorrhoidal banding: a warning. Dis Colon Rectum 28:291–293.
45. Wright AD (1950) Complications of rectal injections. Proc R Soc Med 43:263–266.
46. Marshall JJ (1995) Technical proficiency of trainees performing colonoscopy: a learning curve. Gastrointest Endosc 42:287.
47. Damore LJ, Rantis PC, Vernava AM, Longo WE (1996) Colonoscopic perforations. Dis Colon Rectum 39:1308–1314.
48. Habr-Gama A, Waye JJ (1989) Complications and hazards of gastrointestinal endoscopy. World J Surg 13:193–201.
49. Christie JP, Marrazzo J (1991) Mini-perforation of the colon – not all post-polypectomy perforations require laparotomy. Dis Colon Rectum 34:132–135.
50. Waye JD (1981) The postpolypectomy coagulation syndrome. Gastrointest Endosc 27:184 only.
51. Husson R (1994) Gastroenterologists in trouble. J Med Defence Union 1:4–5.
52. Garbay JR, Suc B, Rotman N, Fourtanier G, Escat J (1996) Multicentre study of surgical complications of colonoscopy. Br J Surg 83:42–44.
53. Thomson SR, Fraser M, Stupp C, Baker LW (1994) Iatrogenic and accidental colon injuries – what to do? Dis Colon Rectum 37:496–502.
54. Maglinte DD, Strong RC, Strate RW (1982) Barium enema after colorectal biopsy; experimental data. Am J Radiol 139:693–697.
55. Morse RM, Spimak JP, Resnich MI (1988) Iatrogenic colon and rectal injuries associated with urological intervention: report of 14 patients. J Urol 40:101–103.
56. Symonds EM (1985) Medico-legal aspects of the therapeutic abortion In: Chamberlain GVP, Orr CJB, Sharp F (eds) Litigation in obstetrics and gynaecology. Proceedings of the Fourteenth Study Group of the RCOG, London, pp 123–129.
57. Patterson DE, Zincke H (1984) Perioperative complications of pelvic lymphadenectomy and radial suprapubic prostatectomy for stage C and D1 prostatic cancer. Urology 23:243–247.
58. Loffer FD, Pent D (1975) Indications, contraindications and complications of laparoscopy. Obstet Gynecol Surg 30:407–427.
59. McMahon AJ, Baxter JN, O'Dwyer PJ (1993) Preventing complications of laparoscopy. Br J Surg 80:1593–1594.
60. Rodrigues-Netto N, Lemos GC, Fiuza JL (1988) Colon perforation following percutaneous nephrolithotomy. Urology 32:223–224.
61. Schofield PF (1989) Clinical features of radiation bowel disease. In: Schofield PF, Lupton EW (eds) The causation and clinical management of pelvic radiation disease. Springer, London p 61–68.
62. Kjorstad KE, Martimbeau PW, Iversen T (1983) Stage 1B carcinoma of the cervix, the Norwegian Radium Hospital: results and complications. Gynecol Oncol 15:42–47.
63. Smith v. Tunbridge Wells Health Authority (1994) 5 Med LR 334
64. Sidaway v. The Royal Bethlem Hospital (1985) 1 All ER 643 HL.
65. Keighley MRB, Williams NS (1993) Impaired sexual function In: Keighley MRB, Williams NS (eds) Surgery of the anus, rectum and colon. Saunders, London pp 268–287.
66. Condon RE (1990) Appendicitis. In: Moody FG (ed) Surgical treatment of digestive disease. Year Book, Chicago, pp 719–739.
67. Bothwell WN, Bleicher RJ, Dent TL (1994) Prophylactic ureteral catheretization in colonic surgery. Dis Colon Rectum 37:330–334.
68. James C (1997) Ureteric damage not always negligent. J Med Defence Union 13:10–11.
69. Brudenell M (1996) Medico-legal aspects of ureteric damage during abdominal hysterectomy. Br J Obstet Gynaecol 103:1180–1183.
70. Leff RG, Shapiro SR (1979) Lower extremity complications of the lithotomy position: prevention and management. J Urol 122:138–139.
71. Stoodley NG, Thomson WHF (1989) Compartment syndrome: a cautionary tale. Br J Surg 76:1296.
72. Bergqvist D, Bohe M, Ekelund G et al. (1990) Compartment syndrome after prolonged surgery with leg supports. Int J Colorect Dis 5:1–5.
73. Peters P, Baker SR, Leopold PW, Taub NA, Burnand KG (1994) Compartment syndrome following prolonged pelvic surgery. Br J Surg 81:1128–1131.
74. Wilsher v. Essex Area Health Authority (1988) 1 All ER 871 HL.
75. Burke J (1961) Effective period of preventive antibiotic action in experimental excisions and dermal lesions. Surgery 50:161–168.

76. Irvin TT, Stoddard CJ, Greaney MG, Duthie HL (1977) Abdominal wound healing: prospective clinical study. Br Med J 2:351.
77. Verstraete M (1997) Prophylaxis of venous thromboembolism. Br Med J 314:123–125.
78. Drug and Therapeutics Bulletin (1992) Preventing and treating DVT. Drug Ther Bull 30:9–12.
79. Kalodiki E, Nicolaides AN (1997) Prevention and treatment of thromboembolism in general surgery. Clin Risk 3:75–79.
80. Rappaport W, Haynes K (1990) The retained surgical sponge following abdominal surgery. Arch Surg 125:405–409.
81. Summerton N (1996) Defensive medical practice. J Med Dental Defence Union 12:8–9.
82. McQuade JS (1991) The medical malpractice crisis – reflections on the alleged causes and proposed cures: discussion paper. J R Soc Med 84:408–411.

9 Treatment of Haemorrhoids

E.A. Carapeti and R.K.S. Phillips

Introduction

Over the years there have been many so-called advances in the treatment of haemorrhoids so that there are now many options for their treatment (Table 9.1). The variety of treatments highlights a lack of consensus, choice often depending on an individual surgeon's experience and expertise rather than evidence. As most are carried out in out-patients, the role for surgery which hereto has required a moderately long hospital stay and time off work has been questioned. However, the evidence in favour of these treatments is mainly from uncontrolled studies and there are few controlled trials with long-term follow-up. In this chapter we look critically at the literature and examine some of the more important studies published over the past 20 years in an attempt to formulate an evidence-based and rational approach to the treatment of this most common anal condition. We then look at day-case haemorrhoidectomy, which is now feasible for all patients fit for day surgery, and which has a very low complication rate and high patient satisfaction whilst being economical.

Non-surgical Treatments for Haemorrhoids

Injection Sclerotherapy

Injection of 5% phenol in almond or arachis oil has been commonly used to treat first- and second-degree haemorrhoids for many decades. Despite its widespread popularity there are few randomised trials and follow-up has been short. These

Table 9.1. Options available for treatment of haemorrhoids

1. Dietary advice, bulk laxatives
2. 5% Phenol injection (sclerotherapy)
3. Barron's band ligation
4. Infrared photocoagulation
5. Bipolar diathermy, electrocoagulation
6. Cryotherapy
7. Manual anal dilatation
8. Lateral sphincterotomy
9. Haemorrhoidectomy

studies have shown phenol injection to be of minor benefit and in the short term only. For example, a small prospective randomised study by Senapati and Nicholls[1] showed phenol injection to be no better than bulk laxatives at 6 months. Similarly, in a 4-year follow-up of 189 patients treated with high-dose phenol injection, Santos et al.[2] found only 42% of patients had been cured or improved whilst the remainder were unchanged (19%), had deteriorated (31%) or needed surgery (9%). In a much smaller study of only 36 patients, Sim et al.[3] found sclerotherapy to be significantly inferior to rubber banding after 3 years when treating first- and second-degree piles. Indeed, a meta-analysis of haemorrhoidal treatments by McRae and McLeod[4] showed that in almost every controlled trial, phenol injection was inferior to all other treatments despite having an acceptable low complication rate.

It is clear from the literature that phenol injection is an ineffective long-term measure for the treatment of even minor piles. It is no more effective than dietary fibre, which in turn seems no more effective than placebo.[5] Anal canal bleeding associated with proctoscopic appearance of first-degree piles is often self-limiting and requires no specific treatment other than dietary advice and to avoid straining. Injection of phenol has been shown by Adami et al.[6] to be associated with bacteraemia in 8% patients, although septicaemic complications are rare. Furthermore, serious urological complications such as impotence, haematuria and urinary clot retention have been reported following inadvertent prostatic injection of phenol.[7] Although complications of injection are rare, when considered in the light of the evidence suggesting its poor clinical effect, its widespread use must be questioned in clinical practice.

Rubber Band Ligation (RBL)

Application of Barron's bands to the base of the pile or to the mucosa above the pile (the "hitch-up" method) is a popular out-patient method for treatment of haemorrhoids. Evidence suggests that it is an effective initial treatment for a proportion of symptomatic internal haemorrhoids. In a recent paper, Bayer et al.[8] reported their 12-year experience of treating haemorrhoids with RBL and showed a 79% cure rate in 2934 patients, although multiple treatment sessions were required by nearly all the patients. Similarly, Alemdaroglu and Ulualp[9] in their 2-year follow-up of 49 patients with bleeding internal piles treated with single-session banding reported 94% "satisfactory" results. Indeed, banding has been shown to be superior to sclerotherapy immediately and at long-term follow-up.[3] By contrast, in a randomised controlled trial Cheng et al.[10] showed banding to be inferior to haemorrhoidectomy in curing piles, despite its superiority over anal dilatation and sclerotherapy. Nevertheless they recommended RBL as a treatment of choice because of the long in-patient stay and higher complication rate after haemorrhoidectomy. Table 9.2 is a summary of results of selected recent controlled trials of haemorrhoidal treatments that report a follow-up of a minimum of 6 months.

Rubber band ligation is not without complications. In a large series of cases treated by RBL over a 7-year period, Bat et al.[17] reported a 2.5% hospitalisation rate (for massive bleeding, urinary retention, prolapsed thrombosed piles, severe sepsis and abscess formation) and 4.6% "minor" complications (minor bleeding, local induration and infection, priapism, slipping of bands, mucosal ulceration and difficulty in urination). The reported incidence of pain after banding varies between 5% and 30% and may be related to the number of piles banded in a

Table 9.2. Recent controlled trials of haemorrhoidal treatments which report a minimum of 6 months follow-up

Reference	Year	No. of patients	Treatments compared	Degree of piles treated	Mean. follow-up (months)	Percentage asymptomatic (% improved)
Murie et al.[11]	1980	100		2–3	12	
		50	RBL			79
		50	Haemorrhoidectomy			98
Cheng et al.[10]	1981	120		2	12	
		30	Injection			60
		30	RBL			83
		30	MAD			80
		30	Haemorrhoidectomy			97
Sim et al.[3]	1983	36		1–2	36	
		18	Injection			22
		18	RBL			76
Templeton et al.[12]	1983	137		1–2	12	
		71	RBL			53 (92)
		66	Infrared			57 (85)
Gartell et al.[13]	1985	269		1–3	32	
		134	Injection			17 (70)
		135	RBL			36 (89)
Senapati et al.[1]	1988	41		PR bleed	6	
		21	Injection			57
		20	Sterculia			47
Hinton et al.[14]	1990	50		3	?	
		24	Bipolar diathermy			83
		26	DC therapy			77
Walker et al.[15]	1990	200		1–3	12 & 48	
		100	Infrared			25–42
		100	RBL/injection			20–39
Randall et al.[16]	1994	100		1–2	12	
		50	Bipolar diathermy			71
		50	DC therapy			66

RBL, rubber band ligation; MAD, manual anal dilatation; DC, direct current.

single session.[18-22] A closer look at many reports reveals more serious complications as well as fatalities associated with RBL. These may be rare, but they highlight the problems associated with a procedure perceived by many as risk-free.[23] There are case reports of fatalities after RBL from haemorrhage,[24] as well as bacterial septicaemia and toxaemia[22,25] and severe pelvic cellulitis.[22,26,27] These reports have occasionally led to debates about safety and appropriateness of RBL as a treatment so widely practised by all grades of surgeons. However, it must be stressed that deaths and serious complications following RBL are rare and the procedure is generally safe and in the short term at least, effective.

On the other hand there are very few studies with long-term data on the treatment of advanced or external (third- and fourth-degree) haemorrhoids with RBL. The evidence here suggests that RBL is often a "holding measure" to be used for patients otherwise medically unfit for surgery.[28] Long-term follow-up often shows recurrence of symptoms and a common course of repeated visits to the surgeon with multiple banding sessions temporarily to control symptoms. The meta-analysis by Mac-Rae and McLeod[29] showed RBL to be inferior to haemorrhoidectomy at curing all grades of haemorrhoids but nevertheless went on to recommend it as the initial choice of treatment because of low complication rates and its feasibility as an out-patient treatment. Even though RBL is commonly performed on out-patients, a prospective questionnaire by Hardwick et al.[30] found RBL caused pain in 84% patients in the first 24 hours (severe in 18%), 60% in the second 24 hours (14% severe), with the overall result that, 28% of patients were unable to return to normal activities. This is important when comparing various treatments with haemorrhoidectomy, as the choice is often based on the out-patient nature of alternative treatments when in fact the post-procedure course may be very different from that expected, to such an extent that Hardwick et al.[30] suggest "informed consent should be obtained before RBL and that patients should be given the opportunity to delay treatment if they so wish".

Infrared Coagulation

This consists of application of an infrared probe to the base of the pile, just proximal to the pile itself, which allows "spot welding" of the pile base using three to five exposures of about 1.5 seconds each to the mucosa. There is usually no need for local anaesthesia and proponents claim immediate return to normal activity. In a meta-analysis, Johanson and Rimm[31] found infrared coagulation to be safe and well tolerated and because of this recommended it above other non-surgical modalities. However they clearly showed it to be inferior to rubber band ligation in achieving a cure, and there was no comparison to haemorrhoidectomy. They found recurrences were significantly more frequent after infrared coagulation, and patients were much more likely to need multiple treatments to achieve symptom relief when compared with RBL. Smith[28] in his review of haemorrhoidal treatments suggested infrared may be useful for minor anal canal bleeding from first- and small second-degree piles as an alternative to sclerotherapy or banding, but for any degree of prolapse such as large second-degree piles or more advanced haemorrhoids they advocated surgery as the preferred option. Similarly, Walker et al.,[15] in a randomised study of 200 patients, found 54% recurrence of prolapse in patients treated with infrared coagulation compared with 27% with RBL after 1 year, with significantly more patients requiring multiple treatments in the infrared group, despite a lower incidence of pain. No differences were found between treatments in patients with non-prolapsing haemorrhoids. These findings are echoed in the meta-analysis by MacRae and McLeod[29], who also looked at the results of haemorrhoidectomy. Patients treated with sclerotherapy or infrared coagulation were more likely to require multiple treatments compared with RBL or haemorrhoidectomy, with the latter being superior to all other modalities despite having a higher complication rate.

There are no reports that take into account the cost of infrared coagulation equipment, maintenance costs, nor the cumulative cost of repeated out-patient visits and multiple treatments required per individual patient. These must be taken into consideration when deciding which of the many treatments available for piles is the best long-term option.

Cryotherapy

This is the application of a liquid nitrogen or nitrous oxide cryoprobe to the mucosa of the haemorrhoid via a bivalve speculum until the surface is frosted. It is probably fair to say that cryotherapy has fallen out of favour with both physicians and patients, and it is no longer in common practice.[32]. First used in the latter half of the 1960s, it was later seen as a promising option by many, based on reports of a few uncontrolled series.[33,34] As with other-non surgical treatments, there are few data from controlled studies. However, long-term reviews have revealed a different picture. A 6-year review of patients treated with cryotherapy by Irving and Walker[35] showed that 40% patients considered cryotherapy "unpleasant" or "extremely unpleasant", whilst at 6 years only 27% patients remained asymptomatic. Of the remainder, 24% considered their symptoms moderate or severe. In addition, even its proponents recommended it for internal and non-prolapsing piles only, as the results are unsatisfactory and the procedure is poorly tolerated for prolapsing and external piles.[36]

Even cryotherapy is not without problems and there are reports of complications and fatalities.[37] The paper by Oh[33] on 7 years' experience of 1000 "cryohaemorrhoidectomies" reported that two-thirds of patients complained of pain from the procedure (mild to severe), and those being treated for prolapsing piles had an unpleasant anal discharge. Similarly Tanaka[38] reported 5% incidence of significant haemorrhage after cryosurgery. Considering the poor results and the significant complication rate, it is no surprise that Ferguson[39] describes cryotherapy as a "fading alternative" in the treatment of haemorrhoids.

Bipolar Diathermy and Direct Current Electrocoagulation

The principle of these procedures is similar to infrared coagulation; tissue destruction by heat. Out-patient treatment is carried out without anaesthesia. Success rates of 80% and higher have been reported in a few uncontrolled studies and it is claimed that the procedures are safe and well tolerated. However, a prospective evaluation by Yang et al.[40] showed that in order to achieve symptom relief, multiple treatment sessions are required, there is associated pain in 20%, rectal ulceration in up to 24%, and occasional significant haemorrhage. In a prospective randomised comparison of bipolar versus direct current electrocoagulation, Randall et al.[16] reported up to 34% recurrent rates and up to 20% rebleeding at 1 year, despite this concluding that both procedures were effective treatments for first- and second-degree haemorrhoids. Longer follow-up data are not available for these procedures and there are few or no data on treatment of advanced haemorrhoids. A randomised comparison of early results of direct current (dc) coagulation with phenol sclerotherapy by Varma et al.[41] showed dc coagulation to have even lower success rate than injection in relieving symptoms, whilst being more tedious, taking significantly longer to perform and having a higher post-procedure discomfort. Again no long-term data are available. In addition there are no controlled trials comparing diathermy and electrocoagulation with the more established treatments such as RBL or haemorrhoidectomy.

Surgical Treatments for Haemorrhoids

Manual Anal Dilatation and Lateral Internal Sphincterotomy

These treatments although still practised by some, were more popular two to three decades ago, and are now widely regarded as outdated treatments for piles.

However, they are still performed by some to reduce postoperative pain after haemorrhoidectomy and in the emergency management of strangulated haemorrhoids. The rationale is the observation that as a group haemorrhoids are associated with a high resting anal sphincter pressure, although a causal relation has never been demonstrated. Although there are many reports of successful outcome after these procedures,[42,43] nevertheless it was evident as early as 1975 that anal dilatation is inferior to haemorrhoidectomy and associated with a higher rate of significant complications especially notably faecal incontinence.[44] Addition of anal dilatation or lateral sphincterotomy to haemorrhoidectomy has been advocated for relief of postoperative pain.[45] However, there are now abundant data to suggest that any analgesic effect is slight and short-lived, but complications, usually of incontinence, are real and sometimes devastating so that neither anal dilatation nor sphincterotomy can be recommended.[46,47]

Haemorrhoidectomy

Surgical excision of haemorrhoids is one of the oldest treatments for piles and is also the most effective. Despite the advent of new techniques, haemorrhoidectomy has remained the only effective long-term cure for external piles. There are several described operations that aim to ligate and excise the haemorrhoid together with any external component. It is probably fair to say that no individual operation has been shown clearly to be best and good results can be obtained from a number of different techniques. The ligation/excision technique of Milligan and Morgan is a safe and well-tried operation which leaves an open wound at the site of the pile. It is the technique most favoured in the UK. The closed haemorrhoidectomy technique described by Ferguson involves primary closure of the wounds with absorbable sutures. It is the most widely practised operation for piles in North America[48] and proponents claim reduced postoperative pain, although this is debated and there is no conclusive evidence for this claim. The submucosal haemorrhoidectomy with a high ligation of the pile pedicle described by Parks is less commonly practised today. More recently diathermy excision of haemorrhoids[49] has grown in popularity, and laser haemorrhoidectomy has been assessed in some centres.

There are few studies comparing Milligan–Morgan haemorrhoidectomy with the closed Ferguson technique. Proponents of the latter suggest that primary closure of the wounds decreases postoperative pain after haemorrhoidectomy. However a survey by Wolfe et al.[50] of surgical practices among North American surgeons showed that closed haemorrhoidectomy was not associated with reduced postoperative pain, fewer complications or shorter hospital stay and earlier return to work. Similarly in a prospective study Roe et al.[51] showed no difference in postoperative pain between the open and closed techniques. Anal sensation was better preserved after submucosal haemorrhoidectomy but this was not reflected in improved function. The two procedures were comparable in other aspects.

A randomised trial comparing diathermy haemorrhoidectomy with the standard Milligan–Morgan technique by Seow-Choen et al.[52] found significantly less use of postoperative analgesics after diathermy excision despite no differences in the severity of pain reported. In addition, the diathermy technique was significantly faster to perform and allowed pedicle ties to be avoided. In another smaller study of 20 patients randomised to diathermy haemorrhoidectomy and scissor excision Andrews et al.[53] found no differences between the two techniques, which were comparable in every aspect.

Laser Haemorrhoidectomy

Lasers have been used to treat haemorrhoids for over 15 years, either as an alternative to the blade or knife as a dissecting instrument or as a device to destroy haemorrhoidal tissue. Iwagaki et al.[54] in a retrospective review reported results of treatment of 1816 consecutive patients with haemorrhoids by applying a CO_2 laser to the pile to destroy it. They claimed favourable results with respect to postoperative pain and relief of symptoms. However, no mention was made of adverse effects, recurrences or costs of treatment, and no comparison made with other more established treatments. Similarly Hodgson and Morgan[55] reported results of laser haemorrhoidectomy under local anaesthesia and intravenous sedation in 90 patients, the majority of whom had second- or third-degree piles. They also claimed favourable results, with all but three patients' wounds healing within 4 weeks and no major complications. They suggested that laser haemorrhoidectomy may simplify management of piles in selected patients. However, no long-term data were given and again no comparison made with other treatments. In a randomised prospective study of laser excision versus closed Ferguson haemorrhoidectomy in 88 patients, Wang et al.[56] reported a surprisingly high incidence of urinary retention after the Ferguson technique (39%) compared with laser haemorrhoidectomy (7%), as well as a significantly higher use of opiate analgesia. But they found no differences in overall complications and healing was significantly slower after laser haemorrhoidectomy.

Many of the early and uncontrolled studies led to the suggestion by some proponents that laser haemorrhoidectomy was a superior alternative to conventional surgery with regards to postoperative pain, healing and safety, whilst being an equally effective cure for piles. However, probably a truer picture is revealed after reviewing the few randomised controlled trials and these suggest a different story. In 1993, Senagore et al.[57] randomised 86 patients for haemorrhoidectomy using the closed Ferguson technique or the Nd:YAG laser. They showed no differences between the two techniques with regards to effectiveness, safety or complications, except for a higher incidence of wound inflammation and dehiscence with laser surgery after 10 days. In addition, laser haemorrhoidectomy was $480 more expensive per case than the Ferguson method with an overall cost excess of $15 360 in the laser group. Similarly Leff[58] in a 3-year comparison of laser versus conventional haemorrhoidectomy in 226 patients found no differences between the two techniques, whilst in a review of treatment modalities for haemorrhoids Smith[59] suggested equipment and maintenance cost as a major disadvantage of laser haemorrhoidectomy, which offered no advantages over conventional techniques.

Future Considerations

Day-case Haemorrhoidectomy

Critical review of the literature suggests that haemorrhoidectomy is still the best treatment for large internal piles and the only effective one for external piles.

However, haemorrhoidectomy causes pain and there is much anxiety among patients and their doctors regarding postoperative pain and return to normal bowel habit. In addition, as with any other procedure there are complications which, although uncommon, have been documented comprehensively. These factors have resulted in this relatively minor operation remaining largely an in-patient procedure despite day surgery being accepted as the best option for many other often more major procedures. However, the various fears and imagined problems can be addressed such that full three-quadrant haemorrhoidectomy is now feasible as an out-patient procedure when a meticulous operative technique and a carefully planned perioperative care package is employed. Patient anxiety is reduced through preoperative consultation when questions are answered, the operation and postoperative recovery carefully explained, and a comprehensive information booklet supplied, as often patients retain only a fraction of the information given at first consultation.

Pain after haemorrhoidectomy can be either defecatory pain due to passage of hard stool, or constant background pain due to a variety of possible factors such as presence of a wound in a richly innervated area, anal sphincter spasm, possible colonisation or infection by bacteria or iatrogenic injury to the internal anal sphincter.[60,61] In order to reduce postoperative constipation and thus defecatory pain, patients can be given a course of lactulose or similar stool softener starting a few days before surgery and continuing for 14 days after. This has been shown in a randomised placebo-controlled study by London et al.[62] significantly to reduce defecatory pain after haemorrhoidectomy. Surgical technique may also influence pain and as diathermy haemorrhoidectomy provides good haemostasis it means that a postoperative anal pack can be avoided. Anal packs are extremely uncomfortable and they may well be the reason why some patients develop urinary retention. Other potential advantages of diathermy haemorrhoidectomy are the excellent visualisation of the operative field and the lack of a pedicle ligature, which can at times incorporate fibres of the internal anal sphincter causing spasm and pain.

To reduce background pain after haemorrhoidectomy various pharmacological strategies can be employed. Operative local infiltration with bupivacaine provides initial pain relief but not prolonged analgesia.[63] Use of non-steroidal anti-inflammatory drugs (NSAIDs) in day surgery is well established,[64] and trials have shown these agents to be as effective as opiates in treating pain after haemorrhoidectomy, whilst being associated with significantly fewer side effects such as urinary retention.[65] NSAIDs should be started intraoperatively (either as a suppository or an intersphincteric injection) and continued as a regular course orally in the postoperative period in preference to opiates. Another strategy may be to produce a reversible "chemical sphincterotomy" by topical application of glyceryl trinitrate (GTN). This has been shown to relieve sphincter spasm and pain associated with anal fissures,[66,67] and may be a useful adjunct to the various measures already mentioned in reducing postoperative pain after haemorrhoidectomy, although to date there are no randomised controlled data to suggest this is really so. Another pharmacological approach is the use of antibiotics. We have recently shown in a double-blind randomised controlled trial that a course of oral metronidazole significantly reduces the secondary pain rise on days 4–7 after day-case haemorrhoidectomy, as well as allowing earlier return to work and resulting in higher patient satisfaction (Carapeti EA, Kamm MA, McDonald PJ, Phillips RKS; Lancet in press). We advocate inclusion of a 7- day course of this antibiotic in the perioperative care package for day-case haemorrhoidectomy.

Table 9.3. Suggested perioperative care package for day-case haemorrhoidectomy

1. Consultation supplemented by information booklet
2. Lactulose (20 ml bid), starting 2 days preoperatively, continued for 2 weeks
3. Diathermy haemorrhoidectomy under general anaesthetic with local infiltration (20 ml 0.25% bupivacaine + adrenaline)
4. No "pedicle ties" and no anal canal dressing
5. Diclofenac suppository (100 mg) at operation
6. Patients discharged home when fully recovered from anaesthetic
7. Diclofenac 50 mg tid for 1 week (or nefopam)
8. Glyceryl trinitrate (GTN) 0.2% topical ointment tid for 1–2 weeks
9. Metronidazole 400 mg tid for 7 days
10. Co-dydramol (paracetamol 500 mg + dihydrocodeine 10 mg) as required
11. Contact number for enquiries or in case of emergency
12. Early out-patient appointment (7–10 days)

Table 9.4. Suggested management strategy for haemorrhoids

Anal canal bleeding
    Appropriate tests to rule out more serious pathology
    Reassurance
    If pressed, injection sclerotherapy

Piles with external component/skin tags
    Day-case haemorrhoidectomy with perioperative oral metronidazole for 7 days

Significant symptomatic internal haemorrhoids without external component
    (a) If after due discussion patient accepts then haemorrhoidectomy as above is probably the best long-term option
    (b) Rubber band ligation is a useful short- to medium-term alternative in those not willing to have a haemorrhoidectomy.

A perioperative care package incorporating the above strategies (Table 9.3) allows haemorrhoidectomy to be performed as a day-case procedure with a low (5%) readmission rate, few complications (comparable to in-patient haemorrhoidectomy) and high patient satisfaction (Carapeti et al; Lancet in press). On a satisfaction scale of 3 (extreme dissatisfaction) to +3 (extreme/complete satisfaction), patients randomised to metronidazole and undergoing day-case haemorrhoidectomy scored an average +2 (very happy to have had day surgery). This means that the best treatment for haemorrhoids is now available without the need for in-patient beds, making it very economical in the long term.

Summary

Many so-called advances and modern treatments for haemorrhoids are inadequate measures in the long term. The authors' current views are set out in Table 9.4. Anal canal bleeding associated with proctoscopic finding of "first-degree piles" is often a self-limiting problem and no specific measures are needed other than exclusion of a more serious proximal pathology and dietary advice in order to prevent constipation and excessive straining. Rubber band ligation (RBL) is an effective treatment for some larger internal piles and can be considered as a first-line option for these, so long as the patient is aware that in the longer term further treatment is likely to become necessary. As treatment failures are frequent, and as repeated visits to out-patient clinics for further treatment are a common experience of many surgeons, patients with internal haemorrhoids who fail RBL (or who, being adequately informed, decide against it) as well as those with external haemorrhoids should now be treated with day-case haemorrhoidectomy as the procedure of choice. Perioperative oral metronidazole should be used as a routine. There is at present little evidence to advocate instead the continued use of any of the other so-called modern techniques of treatment for haemorrhoids reviewed above.

References

1. Senapati A, Nicholls RJ (1988) A randomised trial to compare the results of injection sclerotherapy with a bulk laxative alone in the treatment of bleeding haemorrhoids. Int J Colorectal Dis 3:124–126.
2. Santos G, Novell JR, Khoury G, Winslet MC, Lewis AA (1993) Long-term results of large-dose, single-session phenol injection sclerotherapy for hemorrhoids. Dis Colon Rectum 36:958–961.
3. Sim AJ, Murie JA, Mackenzie I (1983) Three-year follow-up study on the treatment of first and second degree hemorrhoids by sclerosant injection or rubber band ligation. Surg Gynecol Obstet 157:534–536.
4. MacRae HM, McLeod RS (1995) Comparison of hemorrhoidal treatment modalities. A meta-analysis. Dis Colon Rectum 38:687–694.
5. Broader JH, Gunn IF, Alexander-Williams J (1974) Evaluation of a bulk-forming evacuant in the management of haemorrhoids. Br J Surg 61:142–144.
6. Adami B, Eckardt VF, Suermann RB, Karbach U, Ewe K (1981) Bacteremia after proctoscopy and hemorrhoidal injection sclerotherapy. Dis Colon Rectum 24:373–374.
7. Bullock N (1997) Impotence after sclerotherapy of haemorrhoids: case reports. Br Med J 314:419.
8. Bayer I, Myslovaty B, Picovsky BM (1996) Rubber band ligation of hemorrhoids. Convenient and economic treatment. J Clin Gastroenterol 23:50–52.
9. Alemdaroglu K, Ulualp KM (1993) Single-session ligation treatment of bleeding hemorrhoids. Surg Gynecol Obstet 177:62–64.
10. Cheng FC, Shum DW, Ong GB (1981) The treatment of second degree haemorrhoids by injection, rubber band ligation, maximal anal dilatation, and haemorrhoidectomy: a prospective clinical trial. Aust N Z J Surg 51:458–462.
11. Murie JA, Mackenzie I Sim AJ (1980) Comparison of rubber band ligation and haemorrhoidectomy for second- and third-degree haemorrhoids: a prospective clinical trial. Br J Surg 67:786–788.
12. Templeton JL, Spence RA, Kennedy TL, Parks TG, Mackenzie G, Hanna WA (1983) Comparison of infrared coagulation and rubber band ligation for first and second degree haemorrhoids: a randomised prospective clinical trial. Br Med J Clin Res 286:1387–1389.
13. Gartell PC, Sheridan RJ, McGinn FP (1985) Out-patient treatment of haemorrhoids: a randomized clinical trial to compare rubber band ligation with phenol injection. Br J Surg 72:478–479.
14. Hinton CP, Morris DL 1990 A randomized trial comparing direct current therapy and bipolar diathermy in the out-patient treatment of third-degree hemorrhoids. Dis Colon Rectum 33:931–932.
15. Walker AJ, Leicester RJ, Nicholls RJ, Mann CV (1990) A prospective study of infrared coagulation, injection and rubber band ligation in the treatment of haemorrhoids. Int J Colorectal Dis 5:113–116.
16. Randall GM, Jensen DM, Machicado GA, Hirabayashi K, Jensen ME, You SPE (1994) Prospective randomized comparative study of bipolar versus direct current electrocoagulation for treatment of bleeding internal hemorrhoids. Gastrointest Endosc 40:403–410.
17. Bat L, Melzer E, Koler M, Dreznick Z, Shemesh E (1993) Complications of rubber band ligation of symptomatic internal hemorrhoids. Dis Colon Rectum 36:287–290.
18. Bartizal J, Slosberg PA (1977) An alternative to hemorrhoidectomy. Arch Surg 112:534–536.
19. Lee HH, Spencer RJ, Beart RW Jr (1994) Multiple hemorrhoidal bandings in a single session. Dis Colon Rectum 37:37–41.
20. Marshman D, Huber PJ Jr, Timmerman W, Simonton CT, Odom FC, Kaplan ER (1989) Hemorrhoidal ligation. A review of efficacy. Dis Colon Rectum 32:369–371.

21. Oueidat DM, Jurjus AR (1994) Management of hemorrhoids by rubber band ligation. J Med Liban 42:11–14.
22. Wechter DG, Luna GK (1987) An unusual complication of rubber band ligation of hemorrhoids. Dis Colon Rectum 30:137–140.
23. Russell TR, Donohue JH (1985) Hemorrhoidal banding. A warning. Dis Colon Rectum 28:291–293.
24. Dixon AR, Harris AM, Baker AR, Barrie WW (1988) Fatal hemorrhage following rubber band ligation of hemorrhoids. Dis Colon Rectum 31:156 (letter).
25. O'Hara VS (1980) Fatal clostridial infection following hemorrhoidal banding. Dis Colon Rectum 23:570–571.
26. Scarpa FJ, Hillis W, Sabetta JR (1988) Pelvic cellulitis: a life-threatening complication of hemorrhoidal banding. Surgery 103:383–385.
27. Clay LD III, White JJ Jr, Davidson JT, Chandler JJ (1986) Early recognition and successful management of pelvic cellulitis following hemorrhoidal banding. Dis Colon Rectum 29:579–581.
28. Smith LE (1987) Hemorrhoids. A review of current techniques and management. [Review with 39 references]. Gastroenterol Clin North Am 16:79–91.
29. MacRae HM, McLeod RS (1997) Comparison of hemorrhoidal treatments: a meta-analysis. Can J Surg 40:14–17.
30. Hardwick RH, Durdey P (1994) Should rubber band ligation of haemorrhoids be performed at the initial outpatient visit? Ann R Coll Surg Engl 76:185–187.
31. Johanson JF, Rimm A (1992) Optimal nonsurgical treatment of hemorrhoids: a comparative analysis of infrared coagulation, rubber band ligation, and injection sclerotherapy. Am J Gastroenterol 87:1600–1606.
32. Leff E (1987) Hemorrhoids. Postgrad Med 82:95–101.
33. Oh C (1981) One thousand cryohemorrhoidectomies: an overview. Dis Colon Rectum 24:613–617.
34. Rudd WW (1989) Ligation and cryosurgery of all hemorrhoids. An office procedure. Int Surg 74:148–151.
35. Irving AD, Walker MA (1987) Cryosurgery for haemorrhoids: 6-year review of "cured" patients. J R Coll Surg Edinb 32:267–269.
36. Tajana A, Chiurazzi D, De Lorenzi I [Infrared photocoagulation, cryosurgery and laser surgery in hemorrhoidal disease]. [Review with 33 references] [In Italian]. Ann Ital Chir 66:775–782.
37. Anderson J, Steger A (1984) Fatal meningitis complicating cryosurgery for haemorrhoids. Br Med J Clin Res Ed 288:826.
38. Tanaka S (1989) Cryosurgical treatment of hemorrhoids in Japan. Int Surg 74:146–147.
39. Ferguson EF Jr (1988) Alternatives in the treatment of hemorrhoidal disease. South Med J 81:606–610.
40. Yang R, Migikovsky B, Peicher J, Laine L (1993) Randomized, prospective trial of direct current versus bipolar electrocoagulation for bleeding internal hemorrhoids. Gastrointest Endosc 39:766–769.
41. Varma JS, Chung SC, Li AK (1991) Prospective randomised comparison of current coagulation and injection sclerotherapy for the outpatient treatment of haemorrhoids. Int J Colorectal Dis 6:42–45.
42. De Roover DM, Hoofwijk AG, van Vroonhoven TJ (1989) Lateral internal sphincterotomy in the treatment of fourth degree haemorrhoids. Br J Surg 76:1181–1183.
43. Hiltunen KM, Matikainen M (1992) Anal dilatation, lateral subcutaneous sphincterotomy and haemorrhoidectomy for the treatment of second and third degree haemorrhoids. A prospective randomized study. Int Surg 77:261–263.
44. Hardy KJ, Wheatley IC, Heffernan EB (1975) Anal dilatation and haemorrhoidectomy. A prospective study. Med J Aust 2:88–91.
45. Asfar SK, Juma TH, Ala-Edeen T (1988) Hemorrhoidectomy and sphincterotomy. A prospective study comparing the effectiveness of anal stretch and sphincterotomy in reducing pain after hemorrhoidectomy. Dis Colon Rectum 31:181–185.
46. Mathai V, Ong BC, Ho YH (1996) Randomized controlled trial of lateral internal sphincterotomy with haemorrhoidectomy. Br J Surg 83:380–382.
47. Mortensen PE, Olsen J, Pedersen IK, Christiansen J (1987) A randomized study on hemorrhoidectomy combined with anal dilatation. Dis Colon Rectum 30:755–757.
48. Khubchandani IT (1988) Operative hemorrhoidectomy. Surg Clin North Am 68:1411–1416.
49. Loder PB, Phillips RK (1993) Haemorrhoidectomy. Curr Pract Surg 5:29–35.
50. Wolfe JS, Munoz JJ, Rosin JD (1979) Survey of hemorrhoidectomy practices: open versus closed techniques. Dis Colon Rectum 22:536–538.

51. Roe AM, Bartolo DC, Vellacott KD, Locke-Edmunds J, Mortensen NJ (1987) Submucosal versus ligation excision haemorrhoidectomy: a comparison of anal sensation, anal sphincter manometry and postoperative pain and function. Br J Surg 74:948–951.
52. Seow-Choen F, Ho YH, Ang HG, Goh HS (1992) Prospective, randomized trial comparing pain and clinical function after conventional scissors excision/ligation vs. diathermy excision without ligation for symptomatic prolapsed hemorrhoids. Dis Colon Rectum 35:1165–1169.
53. Andrews BT, Layer GT, Jackson BT, Nicholls RJ (1993) Randomized trial comparing diathermy hemorrhoidectomy with the scissor dissection Milligan–Morgan operation. Dis Colon Rectum 36:580–583.
54. Iwagaki H, Higuchi Y, Fuchimoto S, Orita K (1989) The laser treatment of hemorrhoids: results of a study on 1816 patients. Jpn J Surg 19:658–661.
55. Hodgson WJ, Morgan J (1995) Ambulatory hemorrhoidectomy with CO_2 laser. Dis Colon Rectum 38:1265–1269.
56. Wang JY, Chang-Chien CR, Chen JS, Lai CR, Tang RP (1991) The role of lasers in hemorrhoidectomy. Dis Colon Rectum 34:78–82.
57. Senagore A, Mazier WP, Luchtefeld MA, MacKeigan JM, Wengert T (1993) Treatment of advanced hemorrhoidal disease: a prospective, randomized comparison of cold scalpel vs. contact Nd:YAG laser. Dis Colon Rectum 36:1042–1049.
58. Leff EI (1992) Hemorrhoidectomy – laser vs. nonlaser: outpatient surgical experience. Dis Colon Rectum 35:743–746.
59. Smith LE. Hemorrhoidectomy with lasers and other contemporary modalities. [Review with 93 references]. Surg Clin North Am 72:665–679.
60. La Torre F, Nicastro A, Masoni L, Clarioni A, Montori A (1992) Pain after haemorrhoidectomy. Anus 14:107–109.
61. Watts JM, Bennett RC, Duthie HL, Goligher JC (1965) Pain after hemorrhoidectomy. Surg Gynecol Obstet 1037–1042.
62. London NJ, Bramley PD, Windle R (1987) Effect of four days of preoperative lactulose on posthaemorrhoidectomy pain: results of placebo-controlled trial. Br Med J Clin Res Ed 295:363–364.
63. Chester JF, Stanford BJ, Gazet JC. Analgesic benefit of locally injected bupivacaine after hemorrhoidectomy. Dis Colon Rectum 33:487–489.
64. Justins DM (1992) Postoperative pain: a continuing challange. Ann R Coll Surg Engl 74:78–79.
65. O'Donovan S, Ferrara A, Larach S, Williamson P (1994) Intraoperative use of Toradol facilitates outpatient hemorrhoidectomy. Dis Colon Rectum 37:793–799.
66. Loder PB, Kamm MA, Nicholls RJ, Phillips RK (1994) "Reversible chemical sphincterotomy" by local application of glyceryl trinitrate. Br J Surg 81:1386–1389.
67. Lund JN, Scholefield JH (1997) A randomised, prospective, double-blind, placebo-controlled trial of glyceryl trinitrate ointment in treatment of anal fissure. Lancet 349:11–14.

10 The Management of Anal Fissure

J. Beynon and N.D. Carr

Introduction

Anal fissure is characterised by a split in the skin of the sensitive endoderm of the anal canal, which tends to affect the younger age group with a roughly equal sex incidence. Characteristically patients present complaining of pain, bleeding and occasionally pruritis ani. The history of the pain is typical and almost pathopneumonic of the condition and helps differentiate fissure from other painful anal conditions. The pain is at or just after defecation and lasts for a variable amount of time, which can usually be measured in minutes. It then resolves until the next episode of defaecation. Bleeding of a fresh nature is noted on the paper and mucous discharge may cause pruritis. Classically the pear-shaped fissure is seen in the posterior midline and can easily be missed by an inexperienced observer who does not peel apart gently the anal canal. Apart from the duration of the history, chronicity can be determined by the appearances with the presence of sentinel tag implying a fissure of some duration. In females approximately 10% of fissures are found in the midline anteriorly while this is much less common in the male population. Care must be taken if the fissure is in an unusual position to exclude Crohn's disease, anal canal carcinoma, ulcerative colitis, tuberculosis, HIV and syphilis. Instrumentation is invariably difficult or impossible due to pain and if any doubt exists about diagnosis or aetiology, examination under anaesthetic is indicated.

Pathology

The current theories about the aetiology of fissure fall into two main areas. First, and far more likely, is that fissure is a result of internal anal sphincter (IAS) hypertonia; second that fissure is due to hypoperfusion of the anal mucosa.[1-5]

The vascular theory of aetiology revolves around the observation that there is a relative deficiency of blood vessels posteriorly in the anal canal; this is backed up by doppler flow studies which show a relative hypoperfusion in the anal canal. The hypertonia which is well documented in the IAS may well work such that there is further relative reduction in tissue perfusion which results in fissure. IA sphincterotomy or general anaesthesia results in a reduction in the anal resting tone and an increase in anodermal blood flow.

Treatment of Anal Fissure

Treatment of anal fissure can be categorised as follows:

- Conservative
- Pharmacological
- Anal dilatation
- Sphincterotomy
- Anoplasty

Conservative Treatment of Anal Fissure

Conservative treatment of anal fissure has revolved around the avoidance of constipation and the use of appropriate analgesics. The rationale is that the passage
of hard stool was involved in the initial anal trauma and that the easy passage of
soft stool with analgesia to help reduce IAS spasm will provide optimal conditions for healing. Thus dietary manipulation with the use of high fibre food,
appropriate laxatives and non-constipating analgesics are worth a trial in the
acute stage. Conservative methods used such as increasing fibre in association
with sitz baths have been more effective than local applications of topical preparation though results are variable.[6-8] Local anaesthetic applications alone appear to
be of less benefit than other conservative methods of treatment.

Anal dilators in conjunction with local anaesthetic were at one stage regularly used but studies have reported high relapse rates.[9-11] However, a GP study
used a local preparation Proctosedyl (Rousell, Uxbridge, UK) and reported an
overall healing of 80%.[12] Whereas Gough and Lewis[13] in a study on 82 patients
reported that 43.6% healed using 2% lignocaine and 41.9% if a dilator was also
used.

The conservative treatment of anal fissure can summarised as comprising:

- Bulk fibre supplements
- Laxative
- High-fibre diet
- Topical preparations
- Analgesia

New Pharmacological Methods of Treatment

Over recent years new treatments have been used in anal fissure; these revolve
around local application of pharmacological agents. This has been brought about
by a greater understanding of the physiology and anatomy of the anal canal and
the sphincter complex. Four agents have recently been used in the treatment of
anal fissure:

1. Glycerin trinitrate (GTN)
2. Isosorbide dinitrate (ISDN)

3. Botulinum toxin
4. Nifedipine

Glycerin Trinitrate

The use of GTN has evolved from the recognition that relaxation of the IAS is mediated by the neurotransmitter nitric oxide.[14–18] O'Kelly et al.[17,18] have produced convincing evidence for this in the IAS retrieved from abdominoperineal resection specimens. They found a dose-dependent relationship strongly suggesting that NO is a neurotransmitter mediating neurogenic relaxation of the human IAS.

In the clinical setting Watson et al.[19] in a study on 19 patients used GTN in doses of 0.2–0.8%. In 15 of 19 patients a concentration of greater than 0.2% was needed to reduce maximal anal resting pressure (MARP) by at least 25% and nine fissures had healed by 6 weeks. Six required lateral sphincterotomy (LS) and four were lost to follow-up. Eight of the nine patients required a GTN concentration of 0.3% or more to achieve healing. Sixteen patients were resistant to 0.2% GTN. While Lund et al.[20] in an initial report on 21 patients (16 posterior and five anterior fissures) using 0.2% reported healing in 18 by 6 weeks though four recurred (three healed with a second course). They also observed reductions in MARP over 20 minutes after application of ointment. In a further paper Lund and Scholefield[21] reported their experience in 39 patients with chronic fissure. GTN 0.2% was used and MARP recorded (previous surgery had been performed in seven). MARP was reduced by 20 minutes after application. Healing was observed in 14 by 4 weeks and 33 by 6 weeks. The fissure recurred in five patients, four were treated by a second course. One was treated by sphincterotomy.

Other reports have similarly observed the effects of GTN in IAS relaxation with Guillemoit et al.[22,23] reporting a decrease in resting pressure in the upper anal canal in normal and constipated patients as did Loder et al.[24] using 0.2% ointment in a group of 10 patients.

Bacher et al.[25] randomised 35 patients with acute and chronic fissure to receive either GTN or topical anaesthetic gel. Sixty percent healed in the GTN group (91.6% acute, 12.5% chronic) within 14 days in contrast to the other group where no healing was observed. MARP reduction was observed in 20% as was also a reduction in MSP (11%).

Lund and Scholefield[26] have further investigated this in a randomised trial of 80 patients who received 0.2% GTN ointment or placebo. Following 8 weeks of treatment 68% receiving GTN had healed their fissures while in the placebo group only 8% had healed. Linear analogue pain scores fell in both groups, which was maintained in the GTN group post-treatment but not in the placebo group. MARP fell significantly in the GTN group but not in the placebo group and in addition a consequential rise in laser doppler flowmetry was observed in the anodermal blood flow.

Isosorbide

Isosorbide has also been used to treat fissure, its pharmacological effect again being as a NO donor. Various studies have again been published with Schouten et al.,[27] in an initial paper on 16 patients using ISDN 3-hourly, reporting that 15 fissures healed by 12 weeks though mild transient headaches were experienced in all patients. Later they reported their results in a group of 34 patients with chronic fissure.[28]. All were treated for a minimum of 6 weeks and up to a maximum of 12 weeks. Of the group, 22 underwent manometry and laser doppler studies. They reported that fissure-related pain was resolved in all by 10 days while by 6, 9 and 12 weeks fissures were healed in 14 (41%), 22 (65%) and 30(88%) of patients, respectively. Synchronous significant reductions in MARP were also observed as were increases in anodermal blood flow. Relapse occurred in two patients (7%). Their preparation was a composition of ISDN in lactose (Sigma Chemical, Los Angeles) incorporated in a base consisting of 10% lanoline and 10% liquid paraffin in white soft paraffin wax (10 mg were applied 5 times daily). ISDN is metabolised to isosorbide mononitrate (ISMN), which is an active metabolite with a longer effect.

Manookian et al.[29] retrospectively analysed results of a comparative study of 81 patients of 42 acute and 39 chronic fissures. Preparations included 1% ISDN (n=37), 0.2% GTN (n=38) and 0.5% GTN (n=6). Healing with all preparations occurred in 69% of acute fissures and 54% of chronic fissures with no difference between the individual groups.

Botulinum Toxin

Botulinum toxin (BT)is a potent rapidly acting neurotoxin that has also been used in the treatment of fissure.[30,31] Its action is to prevent the release of acetylcholine from presynaptic nerve terminals and some clinical studies have been performed.

Jost and Schimrigk,[32] treated 12 patients with 0.1% diluted BT 50 units/ml injected into the external anal sphincter (EAS) either side of the fissure. This produced healing in 10 of the 12 patients at 3 months but brief episodes of incontinence have been reported. Reduction in maximum voluntary squeeze pressure (MVSP) was noted on day 5. While Gui et al.[33] reported healing in 8 of 10 patients at 2 months. In a large study of 100 patients healing was reported to have occured in 79 patients at 6 months following injection with BT.[34] Smaller doses of BT were used, i.e. 2.5–5 units injected directly into the EAS.

In a double-masked, placebo-controlled trial of BT in 30 patients Maria et al.[35] reported healing in 73% while at 2 months 87% had symptomatic relief. All their patients received two injections into the IAS (treatment group of 15 patients – 20 units of BT toxin A; controls, 15 patients – received saline). Success was defined as healing of the fissure while symptomatic improvement was defined as the presence of fissure without symptoms. Eleven of 15 in the treatment group and 2 of 15 in the control group healed. MARP decreased by 25% in the treatment group. Of the controls three underwent sphincterotomy, 10 received BT of whom seven healed and three underwent surgery after 2 months.

Nifedipine

Nifedipine is a calcium channel blocking agent which inhibits smooth muscle. It has been suggested, based on evidence of the effect of nifedipine on anorectal motility, that it may have a role in the treatment of anal fissure.[36] In a study on patients with haemorrhoids and/or fissure with age-matched and sex-matched normal controls Chrysos et al.[36] reported a reduction in resting anal pressure of 30% in both groups and also significant reductions in the length of the high-pressure zone, frequency and amplitude of slow waves in both groups. Reductions in the presence, frequency and amplitude of ultraslow waves were only observed in the patient group. Transient headache was reported in three. Unfortunately they made no assessment of the effect of treatment on the symptoms of either haemorrhoids or fissure.

Surgical Treatment for Anal Fissure

Aims and Prerequisites for Surgery

Despite time-honoured conservative measures and the more recent advances in the pharmacokinetics of the IAS, many patients obtain only temporary relief from non-operative measures designed to treat anal fissures, and surgical treatment becomes necessary to relieve severe and disabling pain. In addition, chronic fissures with deep ulceration, fibrotic undermined edges, associated anal polyps, tags and superficial fistulae seldom undergo spontaneous healing and provide another indication for surgery.[37]

The objectives of surgery for anal fissure are largely directed towards achieving a reduction in MARP. It is well documented that the majority of patients with anal fissure have an elevated MARP and that reduction of the same is associated with healing of the fissure and cessation of symptoms.[38-43] Moreover, division of the lowermost half or caudal third of the IAS seems to reduce MARP throughout the whole length of the anal canal[42] and, on the basis of vector volume analysis, this reduction appears to be global and symmetrical.[44]

A reduction in MARP can be accomplished either by anal dilatation (AD) or surgical division of the IAS, namely sphincterotomy. Ultrasonic studies have shown that the former procedure may produce fragmentation of the IAS, with disruption at multiple sites,[45,46], whilst the latter operation plainly produces a single point of division. Sphincterotomy may be performed in the posterior midline (PS), or in the right or left lateral position (LS), depending whether the surgeon is right- or left-handed. Furthermore, the fissure itself and any associated skin tags can be excised at the same time.[37]

Anal dilatation was introduced by Recamier[47] in 1829 and was the mainstay of treating anal fissures for many years.[48-51] There is no doubt that this operation is effective in curing the majority of patients with anal fissures.[48,49,51] Nevertheless, the procedure has fallen into disrepute because it is difficult to perform in a controlled way,[52,53] particularly for the surgical trainee, and may produce troublesome mucofaecal leakage.[49] Moreover, major degrees of anorectal incontinence may occur after AD because the procedure can disrupt the somatic musculature of the anal canal, namely, puborectalis and the external anal sphincter.[54]

Although there had been previous descriptions of sphincterotomy, it was Eisenhammer[55] who introduced this procedure in a systematic way for the treatment of anal fissure. He performed posterior midline division of the caudal half of the IAS together with excision of the fissure. In the belief that this operation was superior to AD, several authors reported their experience of posterior sphinctero-tomy in the surgical management of anal fissures.[56-58] Not withstanding the success of PS in achieving pain relief, this procedure carried the disadvantage of producing a posterior gutter in the anal canal which could led to troublesome faecal leakage[49,59-62] and which was difficult to treat surgically.[63] It was against this background that Eisenhammer modified his approach and introduced LS in 1959 on the basis that it produced less deformity of the anal canal and a lower inci-dence of soiling and anorectal incontinence.[64]

More recently, it has been recognised that some patients with anal fissures do not have an elevated MARP. These are usually young women who have recently undergone childbirth. The fissures are situated anteriorly and MARP may be lower than normal.[13, 65,66] Similarly, patients who have undergone AD or sphinc-terotomy and an adequate reduction in MARP may have residual or recurrent fissure. In this group of patients fissure excision with anoplasty has been resur-rected in order to deal with the problem.[66-68]

Surgical Procedures

Anal Dilatation (AD)

There are many descriptions of this technique, which may be performed manually.[48-51,69] The precise technique and operative position will vary from surgeon to surgeon, but important principles include gentle stretching of the anus in a circumferential manner with pressure applied laterally and then in an antero-posterior plane for a duration of 4 minutes. Watts et al.[49] originally suggested that two fingers of each hand be used, though others suggest six.[69] Maximal AD using four fingers of each hand[50] is not recommended for the treatment of anal fissure. Sohn et al.[52] have described the use of the Eisenhammer anal speculum or a balloon for producing more controlled dilatation of the anus and have reported excellent results with no postoperative incontinence.

Lateral Sphincterotomy (LS)

This operation may be performed using either an open (OLS) or closed (subcuta-neous) technique (CLS).[43,53,57-59,61,62,64,70-73] In the former method, the anal canal is gently dilated using a Parks anal retractor, which is opened just enough to put the internal sphincter on stretch. By pulling the retractor towards the operator, the intersphincteric groove is accentuated. The internal sphincter is then exposed through a small incision centred on the intersphincteric groove. The intersphinc-teric space is entered thus liberating the outer surface of the internal sphincter. The inner surface can be similarly exposed by lifting off the anoderm and subcu-taneous tissues. Under direct vision, which is the great advantage of this tech-nique, the internal sphincter can be carefully divided to the level of the dentate line and not beyond. Great care is needed when dividing the IAS in women in that the length divided is often more extensive than intended.[74]

Some surgeons prefer to use the technique of CLS.[72,75] In this operation the internal sphincter is divided by inserting a cataract or similar-sized knife into the intersphincteric groove with the index finger in the anal canal. The blade is then rotated through 90° so that the sharp surface faces inwards. The internal sphincter is then divided against the index finger taking care not to breach the mucosa.[71,72] Alternatively, the submucosal plane can be entered and the internal sphincter divided in an outwards direction.[73,75]

Posterior Sphincterotomy (PS)

Although this was the original method for internal sphincterotomy,[55] it has largely been abandoned in favour of the lateral approach. Healing times were often prolonged and the procedure produced a posterior gutter in the anal canal or "keyhole deformity" which led to imperfections in anorectal continence.[49,56-62]

Results of Surgery

There is still considerable debate concerning the optimum surgical procedure for anal fissure once conservative methods have failed. Success must be judged on the basis of pain relief and healing, residual or recurrent fissure and effects on anorectal continence.

Pain Relief and Healing

AD is still very effective in the treatment of anal fissures and is associated with a high success rate in terms of pain relief and healing. Watts et al.[49] reported on 99 patients who underwent anal dilatation for the treatment of chronic fissure. Ninety-four percent of patients experienced early pain relief, though 16% of patients had a residual or recurrent fissure. The authors commented that anal dilatation had the advantage of simplicity, brief hospital stay and early return to work. Similarly, Marby et al.[76] reported a success rate of 90% after manual anal dilatation and Sohn et al.[16] found that instrumental dilatation of the anus produced a healing rate of greater than 90%. There are many other reports which support these observations.[48,51,53,57,68,70]

Likewise, LS is successful in achieving a high rate of healing and a low recurrence rate (Table 10. 1) and is being increasingly performed as a day-case

Table 10.1. Healing and recurrence after lateral sphincterotomy (all types)

Series	Year	No.	Healing (%)	Recurrence (%)
Abcarian[77]	1980	150	100	1.3
Keighley[78]	1981	71	100	2.5
Ravicumar[79]	1982	60	97	0
Hsu[80]	1984	89	100	5.6
Walker[62]	1985	100	100	0
Gingold[58]	1987	86	96	3.5
Weaver[81]	1987	39	93	5.1
Khubchandani[82] 1989	420	97	0	
Pernikoff[83]	1994	500	99	2
Oh[68]	1995	1313	95	1.3

basis.[58,84,85] On the basis of uncontrolled, retrospective studies, the results of OLS and CLS appear to be comparable in terms of postoperative complications, pain relief and fissure healing though the type and duration of follow-up differ markedly.[41,48,53,55,57–59,61,64,68,72,73,75,40,84,85] In a substantial retrospective study, Garcia-Aguilar et al.[86] compared the results of surgery in 521 patients who had undergone OLS with 343 in whom CLS had been performed. Results were assessed using a postal questionnaire and the median follow-up was 3 years with a range of 1 to 6 years. Symptoms persisted in 3.4% and 5.3% of patients, respectively. Fissures recurred in 10.9% of patients who had undergone OLS and 11.7% of those who had been subjected to CLS. None of these differences achieved statistical significance. Boulos and Araujo,[38] in a prospective randomised study compared two groups of 14 patients treated by either OLS or CLS. In terms of pain relief, healing and return of bowel function there were no statistically significant differences between the two groups. In a larger randomised study, Kortbeck et al.[87] compared the results of the open and closed methods of sphincterotomy and found that fissure healing was similar in the 54 patients subjected to OLS when compared with the 58 who had undergone CLS (96.6% versus 94.4%, respectively). However, the duration of hospital stay was statistically significantly shorter in the CLS group. It would seem therefore that the method of sphincterotomy employed is one of surgical preference and that comparable results can be anticipated with either method.

In terms of fissure healing and pain relief, comparison between AD and either type of LS has produced conflicting results. In a randomised trial, Marby et al.[76] noted a recurrence rate of 10% in patients who had undergone AD compared with 29% in those who had CLS. By contrast, Hawley[70] noted a recurrence rate of 28% after AD compared with 4% after LS at 6 months follow up. Others too have found LS to be more effective than AD in the treatment of anal fissure.[64,68,75,89]

Residual and Recurrent Fissure

Both AD and LS are associated with a small proportion of fissures which persist or recur. Poor patient selection such as females with coexisting obstetric sphincter injury who have "normotonic" fissures[66] undoubtedly accounts for some of these failures. In addition, Farouk et al.[88] have pointed out that inadequate sphincterotomy may also be the cause of recurrent fissure. These authors examined 13 patients with residual fissure after LS using endoanal ultrasonography. They found that two patients had been subjected to a very limited division of the IAS whilst in the remaining 11 no sphincterotomy had been performed at all. These observations emphasise that all patients with residual or recurrent anal fissures should undergo endoanal ultrasonography and anorectal physiology in order to evaluate sphincter morphology and function prior to further surgery. If MARP remains high or the previous sphincterotomy has been less than adequate, then either completion or contralateral sphincterotomy is appropriate. By contrast, in patients who have low MARPs and/or endosonic evidence of complete sphincterotomy or defects in the external sphincter then fissure excision with anoplasty can produce satisfactory results.[66,67]

Anorectal Incontinence

Imperfections in continence may occur after either AD or sphincterotomy and remain a vexing problem for both patient and surgeon alike. Hoffman and Goligher[75] reported 90 patients who had undergone AD for the treatment of anal fissure. Postoperative soiling of underclothes was noted in 22% of patients, incontinence of flatus in 13% and frank faecal incontinence in 2%. This high incidence of varying degrees of anorectal incontinence has since been echoed by other authors.[89] The advent of endoanal ultrasonography has allowed a better understanding of this problem and it is now recognised that uncontrolled disruption of the IAS and, to a lesser extent, the somatic musculature of the anal canal may occur after AD.[45,46]

Incontinence appears to be less of a problem after LS (Table 10.2) but data are difficult to analyse because of the lack of consistency in the definition of incontinence and the different duration of follow-up of patients between series. Nevertheless, endoanal ultrasonography has once again demonstrated that during the operation of LS, by either method, overzealous division of the IAS may be inapplicably performed[74] and the EAS may also be injured.[88]

The surgical management of incontinence after either AD, PS or LS is difficult.[63] In those patients who have undergone AD who have fragmentation of one or both sphincter mechanisms, postanal repair is unsuccessful in the long term and it remains to be seen whether more sophisticated methods of reconstruction such as stimulated graciloplasty or the insertion of an artificial sphincter will be successful.[93] In those patients with discrete defects of the IAS after either PS or LS, attempts at direct repair of the IAS have uniformly failed because the divided ends of the IAS are difficult to approximate and do not hold sutures well.[94,95] The alternative approach of anoplasty to correct posterior keyhole deformities by inlaying a soft tissue buttress of subcutaneous fat and skin was originally described by Corman[96] and has been successfully used by the present authors to correct defects at other points on the circumference of the anal canal.[95] The injection of collagen into the anal canal in order to increase the contribution of the soft tissues to the fine tuning of anal continence[97,98] has recently been suggested[99] and although short-term results appear excellent longer-term outcome remains unknown.

Table 10.2. Incontinence after lateral sphincterotomy

Series	Year	No.	Incontinence(%)
Abcarian[77]	1980	150	30
Keighley[78]	1981	71	2
Ravicumar[79]	1982	60	5
Hsu[80]	1984	89	0
Jensen[89]	1984	30	0
Walker[62]	1985	100	15
Gingold[58]	1987	86	0
Lewis[90]	1988	50	6
Khubchandani[82]	1989	420	35
Pernikoff[83]	1994	500	8
Oh[68]	1995	1313	1.5
Usatoff[91]	1995	98	18
Hananel[92]	1997	265	1

Anal Fissures in Children

A large proportion of anal fissures seen in neonates and children heal spontaneously with conservative measures, but surgical intervention may be occasionally be required.[100] The threshold for surgery is higher than in adults, but the general principles remain similar. If anal dilatation is selected as the method of treatment great care is required and it is the authors practice to use instrumental dilatation with a nasal speculum. Lateral sphincterotomy may also be performed in children. Cohen et al.[101] studied its use in 23 children ranging from 8 to 168 months of age, and reported a greater than 70% parent–child satisfaction score and healing of the fissure in all children. Nevertheless caution may be required particularly in girls.[102,103]

Summary Points

Recommendations for treatment of anal fissure:

- Full evaluation
- Conservative measures
- Gentle anal dilatation in cases where neuropathy suspected
- LS for most patients
- Anoplasty in resistant cases

References

1. Farouk R, Duthie GS, MacGregor AB, Bartolo DCC (1994) Sustained internal sphincter hypertonia in patients with chronic anal fissure. Dis Colon Rectum 37:424–429.
2. Gibbons CP, Read NW (1986) Anal hypertonia in fissures; cause or effect? Br J Surg 73:443–445.
3. Schouten WR, Briel JW, Auwerda JJA (1994) Relationship between anal pressure and anodermal blood flow. Dis Colon Rectum 37:664–669.
4. Schouten WR, Briel JW, Boerma MO, Auwerda JJA, de Graaf EJR (1996) The ischaemic nature of anal fissure. Br J Surg 83: 63–65.
5. Klosterhalfen B, Vogel P, Rixen H, Mittermayer C (1989) Topography of the inferior rectal artery; a possible cause of chronic, primary anal fissure. Dis Colon Rectum 32:43–52.
6. Jensen SL (1986) Treatment of first episodes of acute anal fissure: prospective randomised study of lignocaine ointment versus hydrocortisone ointment or warm sitz baths plus bran. Br Med J 292:1167–1169.
7. Maldoff RD (1998) Pharmacologic therapy for anal fissure. N Engl J Med 338:257–259.
8. Sharp FR (1996) Patient selection and treatment modalities for chronic anal fissure. Am J Surg 171:512–515.
9. Lock MR, Thomson JP (1977) Fissure-in-ano: the initial management and prognosis. Br J Surg 64:355–358.
10. Fries B, Rietz K-A (1964) Treatment of fissure in ano. Acta Chir Scand 128:312–315.
11. Goivaninetti GD, Manzi M, Marchi L et al. (1986) Use of anal dilators in the conservative therapy of anal rhagades. Chir Ital 38:666–670.
12. A general practitioner study to evaluate the efficacy of 'Proctosedyl' ointment in the treatment of acute fissure-in-ano (1970). Br J Clin Pract 24:289–291.
13. Gough MJ, Lewis A (1983) The conservative treatment of fissure-in-ano. Br J Surg 70:175–176.
14. Rattan S, Sarkar A, Chakder S (1992) Nitric oxide pathway in rectoanal inhibitory reflex of opossum internal anal sphincter. Gastroenterology 103:43–50.
15. Rattan S, Chakder S (1992) Role of nitric oxide as a mediator of internal anal sphincter. Am J Physiol 262: G107–G112.

16. O'Kelly TJ, Davies JR, Brading AF, Mortensen NJMcC (1994) Distribution of nitric oxide synthase containing neurons in the rectal myenteric plexus and anal canal. Morphologic evidence that nitric oxide mediates the rectoanal inhibitory reflux. Dis Colon Rectum 37:350–357.

17. O'Kelly (1996) Nerves that say NO: a new perspective on the human rectoanal inhibitory reflex. Ann R Coll Surg Engl 78:31–38.

18. O'Kelly T, Brading A, Mortensen NJMcC (1993) Nerve mediated relaxation of the human internal anal sphincter: the role of nitric oxide. Gut 34:689–693.

19. Watson SJ, Kamm MA, Nicholls RJ, Phillips RKS (1996) Topical glyceryl trinitrate in the treatment of chronic anal fissure. Br J Surg 83:771–775.

20. Lund JN, Armitage NC, Scholefield JH (1996) Use of glyceryl trinitrate ointment in the treatment of anal fissure. Br J Surg 83:776–777.

21. Lund JN, Scholefield JH (1997) Glyceryl trinitrate is an effective treatment for anal fissure. Dis Colon Rectum 40:468–470.

22. Guillemot F, Leroi H, Lone YC, Rousseau CG (1993) Action of in situ nitroglycerin on upper anal canal pressure of patients with terminal constipation. A pilot study. Dis Colon Rectum 36:372–376.

23. Guillemot F, Lone YC, Leroi H, Lamblin MD, Cortot A (1992) Nitroglycerin in situ reduces upper anal canal pressure. Dig Dis Sci 37:155 (letter).

24. Loder PB, Kamm MA, Nicholls RJ, Phillips RKS (1994) "Reversible chemical sphincterotomy" by local application of glyceryl trinitrate. Br J Surg 81:1386–1389.

25. Bacher H, Mischinger IIJ, Werkgartner G, Cerwenka II, El-Shabrawii A, Pfeifer J (1997) Local nitroglycerin for treatment of anal fissures: an alternative to lateral sphincterotomy? Dis Colon Rectum 40:840–845.

26. Lund JN, Scholefield JH (1997) A randomised, prospective, double-blind, placebo controlled trial of glyceryl trinitrate ointment in the treatment of anal fissure. Lancet 349:11–14.

27. Schouten WR, Briel JW, Boerma MO, Auwerda JJA (1995) Pathophysiological aspects and clinical outcome of intra-anal application of isosorbide dinitrate in patients with chronic anal fissure. Gut 36(Supp 1):A16 (abstract).

28. Schouten WR, Briel JW, Boerma MO, Auwerda JJA, Wilms EB, Graatsma BH (1996) Pathophysiological aspects and clinical outcome of intra-anal application of isosorbide dinitrate in patients with chronic anal fissure. Gut 39:465–469.

29. Manookian CM, Fleshner P, Moore B, Teng F, Cooperman H, Sokol T (1998) Topical nitroglycerin in the management of anal fissure: an explosive outcome. Am Surg 64:962–964.

30. Jankovic J, Brin MF (1991) Therapeutic uses of botulinum toxin. N Engl J Med 324:1186–1194.

31. Ashton AC, Dolly JO (1988) Characterisation of the inhibitory action of botulinum neurotoxin type A in the release of several transmitters from rat cerebrocortical synaptosomes. J Neurochem 50:1808–1816.

32. Jost WH, Schimrigk K (1994) Therapy of anal fissure using botulin toxin. Dis Col Rectum 37:1321–1324.

33. Gui D, Cassetta E, Anastasio G, Bentivoglio AR, Maria G, Albanese A (1994) Botulinum toxin for chronic anal fissure. Lancet 344:1127–1128.

34. Jost WH (1997) One hundred cases of anal fissure treated with Botulin toxin: early and long-term results. Dis Colon Rectum 40:1029–1032.

35. Maria G, Cassetta E, Gui D, Brisinda G, Bentivoglio AR, Albanese A (1998) A comparison of botulinum toxin and saline for the treatment of chronic anal fissure. N Engl J Med 338:217–220.

36. Chrysos E, Xynos E, Tzovaras G, Zoras OJ, Tsiaoussis J, Vassilakis SJ (1996) Effect of nifedipine on rectoanal motility. Dis Colon Rectum 39:212–216.

37. Killingback M. (1988) Anal fissure and fistula with special reference to high fistula. In: DeCosse JJ, Todd IP (eds) Anorectal surgery.Churchill Livingstone, Edinburgh, p 85.

38. Northmann BJ, Schuster MM (1974) Internal anal sphincteric derangment with anal fissures. Gastroenterology 67:216–220.

39. Boulos PB, Araugo JGC (1984) Adequate internal anal sphincterotomy for chronic anal fissure. Br J Surg 71:360–362.

40. McLange M, Colin JF, Van Wymersch T, Vanheuverswyn R (1992) Anal fissure: correlation between symptoms and manometry before and after surgery. Int J Colorectal Dis 7:188–211.

41. Fressa EE, Sandei F, Leoni G, Biral M (1992)Conservative and surgical treatment in acute and chronic anal fissures. A study on 308 patients. Int J Colorectal Dis 7:118–119.

42. McNamara MJ, Percy JP, Fielding IR (1990) A manometric study of anal fissure treatment by subcutaneous internal sphincterotomy. Ann Surg 211:235–238.

43. Prohm P, Bonner C (1995) Is manometry essential for surgery of chronic fissure-in-ano? Dis Colon Rectum 381:735–738.

44. Williams N, Scott NA, Irving MH (1995) Effect of lateral sphincterotomy on internal anal sphincter function. A computerised vector manometric study. Dis Colon Rectum 38:700–704.
45. Sultan AH, Nicholls RJ, Kamm MA, Hudson CN, Beynon J, Bartram CI (1993) Anal endosonography and correlation with in vitro and in vivo anatomy. Brit J Surg 1993; 80:508–511.
46. Speakman CTM, Burnett SJD, Kamm MA, Bartram CI (1991) Sphincter injury after anal dilatation demonstrated by anal endosonography. Br J Surg 78:1429–1430.
47. Recamier JCA (1900) Quotes by Goodsall DA, Miles WE. In: Diseases of the anus and rectum, part 1. Longman Green, London.
48. Graham-Stewart CW, Greenwood RK, Lloyd-Davies RW (1961) A review of 50 patients with fissure in ano. Surg Gynecol Obstet 113:445–448.
49. Watts J, Bennett RC, Goligher JC (1964) Stretching of anal sphincters in the treatment of fissure in ano. Br Med J ii: 342–343.
50. Lord PH (1968) A new regime for the treatment of haemorrhoids. Proc R Soc Med 611:935–939.
51. Hancock RD (1972) The internal sphincter and anal fissure. Br J Surg 64:92–95.
52. Sohn N, Eisenberg M, Weisntein MA, Lugo RN (1992) Precise anorectal sphincter dilatation – it's role in the treatment of anal fissures. Dis Colon Rectum 35:322–327.
53. Saad AM, Omer A (1992) Surgical treatment of chronic fissure in ano: a prospective randomised study. East Afr Med Forum 69:613–615.
54. Neilsen MB, Rasmussen OO, Pedersen JF, Christiansen J (1993) Risk of sphincter damage and anal incontinence after anal dilatation for fissure-in-ano. An endosonographic study. Dis Colon Rectum 36:677–680.
55. Eisenhammer S (1951) The surgical correction of chronic anal (sphincteric) contraction. South Afr Med Forum 25:486–489.
56. Morgan CN, Thompson HR (1956) Surgical anatomy of the anal canal with special reference to the surgical importance of the internal sphincter and conjoint to longitudinal muscle. Ann R Coll Surg Engl 19:88–93.
57. Tzu-Chin-Hsu, Mackeigan JM (1984) Surgical treatment of chronic anal fissure: a retrospective study of 1753 cases. Dis Colon Rectum 27:474–478.
58. Gingold BS (1987) Simple in office sphincterotomy with partial fissuretomy for chronic anal fissure. Surg Gynecol Obstet 165:46–48.
59. Bennett RC, Goligher JC (1962) Results of internal sphincterotomy for anal fissure. Br Med J ii:1500–1503.
60. Bennett RC, Duthie HL (1964) The functional importance of the internal anal sphincter. Br J Surg 51:865–869.
61. Hardy KJ (1967) Internal sphincterotomy: an appraisal with special reference to sequelae. Br J Surg 54:30–31.
62. Walker WH, Rothenberger DA, Goldberg SM (1988) Morbidity of internal sphincterotomy for anal fissure and stenosis. Dis Colon Rectum 28:832–835.
63. Mazier WP (1985) Keyhole deformity: fact or fiction? Dis Colon Rectum 8:8–10.
64. Eisenhammer S (1959) The evaluation of internal anal sphincterotomy – operation with special reference to anal fissure. Surg Obstet Gynaecol 109:583–590.
65. Martin JD (1953) Post partum anal fissure. Lancet I:271–273.
66. Nyam DL, Wilson RG, Stewart KJ, Farouk R, Bartolo DL (1995) Island advancement flaps in the management of anal fissures. Br J Surg 82:326–328.
67. Leong AF, Seow-Choen F (1995) Lateral sphincterotomy compared with anal advancement flap for chronic anal fissure. Dis Colon Rectum 38:69–71.
68. Oh C, Divino CM, Steinhagen RM (1995) Anal fissure: 20-year experience. Dis Colon Rectum 38:378–382.
69. Keighley MRB (1993) Fissure in ano. In: Keighley MRB, Williams NS (eds) Surgery of the anus, rectum and colon. Saunders, London, pp 375–377.
70. Hawley PR (1969) The treatment of chronic fissure in ano. Br J Surg 56:915–918.
71. Notaras MJ (1969) Lateral subcutaneous sphincterotomy for anal fissure – a new technique. Proc R Soc Med 62:713.
72. Notaras MJ (1971) The treatment of anal fissure by lateral subcutaneous internal sphincterotomy – a technique and results. Br J Surg 58:96–100.
73. Bailey RV, Rubins RJ, Salvati EP (1978) Lateral internal sphincterotomy. Dis Colon Rectum 21:584–586.
74. Sultan AH, Kamm MA, Nicholls RJ, Bantram CI (1994) Prospective study of the extent of internal anal sphincter division during internal sphincterotomy. Dis Colon Rectum 37:1031–1033.
75. Hoffman DC, Golighar JC (1970) Lateral subcutaneous sphincterotomy in the treatment of anal fissure.Br Med J iii:673–675.

76. Marby M, Alexander-Williams J, Buchmann P, et al. (1979) A randomised controller to compare anal dilatation with lateral subcutaneous sphincterotomy for anal fissure. Dis Colon Rectum 22:308–311.

77. Abcarian H (1980) Surgical correction of chronic anal fissure: results of lateral sphincterotomy. Dis Colon Rectum 23:31–36.

78. Keighley MRB, Creca F, Nevah E et al. (1981) Treatment of anal fissure by lateral subcutaneous sphincterotomy should be done under general anaesthesia. Br J Surg 68:400–401.

79. Ravikumar TS, Sridhar S, Rao RN (1982) Subcutaneous lateral sphincterotomy for chronic fissure in ano. Dis Colon Rectum 25:789–801.

80. Hsu T, MacKeigan JM (1984) Surgical treatment of chronic anal fissure. Dis Colon Rectum 27:475–478.

81. Weaver RM, Ambrose NS, Alexander-Williams J, Keighley MRB (1987) Manual dilatation of the anus versus lateral subcutaneous sphincterotomy in the treatment of chronic fissure in ano: results of a prospective randomized clinical trial. Dis Colon Rectum 30:420–423.

82. Khubchandani IT, Reed JF (1989) Sequelae of internal sphincterotomy for chronic fissure in ano. Br J Surg 76:431–434.

83. Pernikoff BJ, Eisenstat TE, Rubin RJ, et al. (1994) Reappraisal of partial lateral sphincterotomy. Dis Colon Rectum 37:1291–1295.

84. Hiltunen KM, Matikainen M (1991) Closed lateral subcutaneous sphincterotomy under local anaesthetic in the treatment of chronic anal fissure. Chirurg Gynaecol 80:353–356.

85. Nenfild DM, Param H, Bendaham J, Freund U (1995) Outpatient surgical treatment of anal fissure. Eur Forum Surg 161:435–438.

86. Garcia-Aguilar J, Belmonte L, Long WD, Losory AC, Madoff RD (1996) Open versus closed sphincterotomy for chronic anal fissure: long term results. Dis Colon Rectum 39:440–443.

87. Kartbeck JB, Langevin JM, Kloo RE, Heine JA (1992) Chronic fissure in ano: a randomised study comparing open and subcutaneous lateral internal sphincterotomy. Dis Colon Rectum 35:835–837.

88. Farouk R, Monson JR, Duthie GS (1997) Technical failure of lateral sphincterotomy for the treatment of chronic anal fissure: a study using endoanal ultrasonography. Br J Surg 84:84–85.

89. Jensen SL, Land F, Nielson OV, Tange G (1984) Lateral subcutaneous sphincterotomy versus anal dilatation in the treatment of fissure in ano in outpatients. Br Med J 289:528–530.

90. Lewis TH, Gorman ML, Prager ED, Robertson WG (1988) Long-term results of open and closed sphincterotomy for anal fissure. Dis Colon Rectum 31:368–371.

91. Usatoff V, Polglase AL (1995) The longer term results of internal anal sphincterotomy for anal fissure. Aust NZ J Surg 65:576–578.

92. Hananel N, Gordon PH (1997) Lateral internal sphincterotomy for fissure in ano revisited. Dis Colon Rectum 40:597–602.

93. Vaisey CJ, Kamm MA, Nicholls RJ (1998) Recent advances in the surgical treatment of faecal incontinence. Br J Surg 85:596–603.

94. Leroi AM, Kamm MA, Weber J, Denis P, Hawley PR (1997) Internal anal sphincter repair. Int J Colorectal Dis 12:243–245.

95. Morgan R, Patel B, Beynon J, Carr ND (1997) Surgical management of anorectal incontinence due to internal anal sphincter deficiency. Br J Surg 84:226–230.

96. Corman ML (1983) Anoplasty. In: Todd IP, Fielding LP (eds) Rob and Smith's Operative surgery: alimentary tract and abdominal wall. III. Colon, rectum and anus, 4th edn. Mosby, St Louis, pp 586–592.

97. Gibbons CP, Bannister JJ, Trowbridge GA, Read NW (1986) An analysis of anal sphincter pressure and anal compliance in normal subjects. Int J Colorectal Dis 1:231–237.

98. Gibbons CP, Trowbridge EA, Bannister JJ, Read NW (1988) The mechanics of the anal sphincter complex. J Biomech 21:601–604.

99. Kumar D, Benson M. (1997) GAX collagen injections: a novel treatment for faecal incontinence. Gut 40(Suppl 1):A52.

100. Freeman NV (1993) Miscellaneous paediatric disorders. In: Keighley MRB, Williams NS (eds) Surgery of the anus, rectum and colon. Saunders, London, pp 2426–2427.

101. Cohen A, Dehn TC (1995) Lateral subcutaneous sphincterotomy for treatment of anal fissure in children. Br J Surg 82:1341–1342.

102. Evans DA (1996) Lateral subcutaneous sphincterotomy for treatment of anal fissure in children. Br J Surg 83:571.

103. Turnock RR (1996) Lateral subcutaneous sphincterotomy for treatment of anal fissure in children. Br J Surg 83:424–425.

Index